W9-BWX-887

Cancer with Hope

Cancer
with
Hope

Facing Illness, Embracing Life,
and Finding Purpose

Mike Armstrong
with Eric A. Vohr

Foreword by Theodore DeWeese, MD

JOHNS HOPKINS UNIVERSITY PRESS
Baltimore

Note to the Reader: This book is not meant to substitute for medical care, and treatment should not be based solely on its contents. Instead, treatment must be developed in a dialogue between the individual and his or her physician. The book has been written to help with that dialogue.

© 2021 Johns Hopkins University Press
All rights reserved. Published 2021
Printed in the United States of America on acid-free paper
9 8 7 6 5 4 3 2 1

Johns Hopkins University Press
2715 North Charles Street
Baltimore, Maryland 21218-4363
www.press.jhu.edu

Library of Congress Cataloging-in-Publication Data

Names: Armstrong, Mike, 1938– author. | Vohr, Eric A., author. |
    DeWeese, Theodore L., writer of foreword.
Title: Cancer with hope : facing illness, embracing life, and finding purpose /
    Mike Armstrong ; with Eric A. Vohr ; foreword by Theodore DeWeese,
    MD.
Description: Baltimore : Johns Hopkins University Press, [2021] |
    Includes bibliographical references and index.
Identifiers: LCCN 2020015936 | ISBN 9781421440170 (hardcover) |
    ISBN 9781421440187 (paperback) | ISBN 9781421438382 (ebook)
Subjects: LCSH: Armstrong, Mike, 1938– —Health. | Cancer—
    Patients—United States—Biography. | Cancer—Psychological aspects.
Classification: LCC RC265.6.A36 A3 2021 | DDC 616.99/40092 [B]—dc23
LC record available at https://lccn.loc.gov/2020015936

A catalog record for this book is available from the British Library.

Special discounts are available for bulk purchases of this book. For more informa-tion, please contact Special Sales at specialsales@jh.edu.

Johns Hopkins University Press uses environmentally friendly book materials, including recycled text paper that is composed of at least 30 percent post-consumer waste, whenever possible.

For my wife, Anne
Our daughters, Linda, Julie, and Kristy
and our grandchildren, Nicole, Alex, John, Abigail, Jessica,
Nicky, Austen, Jacqueline, Charlie, and Drew

Mike Armstrong

Contents

Foreword

A diagnosis of cancer is life changing. It is often accompanied by a range of emotions that are as intense and wide-ranging as those associated with any other human experience. Fear, depression, anger, and the uncertainty of what treatment might involve can be all-consuming, and each patient must navigate their way through this labyrinth of new experiences.

In this book, Mike Armstrong provides a vivid description of his own journey following two different cancer diagnoses and the associated treatments, as well as a risky and debilitating breathing condition. I have had the pleasure of knowing Mike for more than fifteen years and have the honor of being his physician for his prostate cancer. I have been treating patients with cancer for more than twenty years and been fortunate to treat thousands of men with prostate cancer, and Mike is, indeed, a unique figure.

When I first met Mike, it was clear he was a very positive, engaging, and motivated man, consistent with his long history as a senior executive of several large corporations. These were the same attributes he brought to the diagnosis and treatment of his prostate cancer. As he describes in his book, we often discussed why he was able to remain so positive and exude a never-stop-fighting attitude. This ability came from the life lessons given to him by his mother and the enduring loving support of his wonderful wife, Anne. I am convinced both were key in allowing Mike to successfully complete his cancer treatment and overcome the rare, debilitating breathing issues that coincidently appeared at the same time. As we discussed his perspective on life, I often thought of a quote attributed to the Roman emperor Marcus Aurelius, which I think sums up Mike's philosophy and source of strength: "You have power over your mind—not outside events. Realize this, and you will find strength."

Never giving up and mustering the strength to slog through adversity on his way to health has provided clarity of purpose and a sense of focus for the balance of Mike's life. Indeed, the power to control those things he can and to let go of those things he cannot is, I believe, part of the explanation for the extraordinary post-cancer life that Mike and Anne have pursued. Together, they have identified programs that would thrive if they directed their attention and resources toward them. With their strength of purpose, Mike and Anne have already changed thousands of lives and are supporting other efforts that are on course to change thousands more.

The underlying themes contained in *Cancer with Hope* reflect a story that could be told by many patients who have cancer. Inner strength and the hope for better health are something I have seen in my patients, and their bravery to face the unknown is both humbling and uplifting to me. When a patient is first diagnosed with cancer, strength and hope may seem elusive. I believe patients newly diagnosed with cancer will find that Mike's book provides a path to recognizing their own inner strength and the spirit to never lose hope, and encourages them to seek support for their journey from those on their team charged with caring for them.

Theodore DeWeese, MD

Cancer with Hope

Prologue

In the 1990s, I was chief executive officer (CEO) of Hughes Electronics, a major US defense contractor that designed, built, and launched some of the world's first geosynchronous satellites. Unlike low-orbit satellites, which are constantly moving in relation to the Earth's surface (spinning around the planet at an altitude of 100 to 1,200 miles), geosynchronous satellites travel about 22,000 miles above the planet and spin with the Earth, maintaining the same position over a designated area of the Earth's surface. These "stationary" satellites were in demand with the military and intelligence agencies, as they provided consistent, accurate, and important strategic information.

Satellite launches are a series of controlled explosions from very powerful rocket engines. These rockets have relatively high reliability. Due to the extremely complex nature of a rocket launch, however, the industry experienced around a 10 percent failure rate for geosynchronous satellite launches during the 1990s.

One of our clients, the United States Navy, had ordered our most advanced surveillance satellite, which cost roughly $350 million to design, build, and launch. On launch day, we all gathered in the Hughes satellite control room with great anticipation to watch the live video of what we hoped would be a successful liftoff. The satellite left the launch pad without issue and soon vanished into the upper atmosphere on its journey into orbit.

Several hours after the launch, Steve Dorfman, the Hughes executive for our satellite division, knocked on the door of my office. I could tell by the expression on his face that something was wrong. He told me the main thruster engines had failed; thus, the satellite had not reached its designated orbit. He explained that the satellite was not damaged, but in its current position it was useless. His team would further assess the situation and determine if we would have to abandon both the satellite and its mission. In that case, our insurance policy would reimburse us for 100 percent of our costs, but we'd lose out on any profit we would have realized had we been able to successfully launch the satellite.

First thing the following morning, I met with Steve and some members of his team to learn about their findings. I fully expected them to confirm that we needed to abandon this satellite, collect the insurance money, and build and launch a new satellite for the Navy.

To my surprise, they suggested something that I had never imagined possible. They said that we could use some of the on-board fuel and positioning jets in the satellite to slowly propel it into the gravitational field of the moon. As the satellite entered the moon's gravity, it would start to "fall" into the moon and accelerate. If all went as planned, the satellite would "slingshot" around the moon and exit the moon's gravitational field with enough inertia to redirect the satellite to its intended position orbiting the Earth. They told me the entire maneuver would use only 25–30 percent of the satellite's fuel. This would reduce the life span of the satellite by roughly one quarter, meaning we could still make a sizeable profit selling it to the Navy for three-quarters of its original price.

Steve cautioned that if we tried this maneuver, we would lose half of the $350 million payout from the insurance company, whether it was successful or not. That would be okay if we pulled it off, because half the insurance money plus what we received from the Navy for the "slightly used" satellite would put us ahead of what we could get if we scrapped it and accepted the full insurance payout. However, if we failed, we'd lose both the satellite and $175 million.

You might have seen spacecraft being hurled around the moon in Hollywood movies, but this was actually the first time a civilian contractor had attempted this kind of thing. Steve assured me that, while the slingshot concept was a technologically sound plan, there were clear risks, which became apparent to me as he walked me through the possible failure points. I had several years of experience working with the Hughes satellite team, and I knew they were some of the best engineers in the world. I reminded Steve that Hughes could lose $175 million if the project failed and that we might just be throwing good money after bad. Steve said he was aware of the risks but thought they were manageable and was confident his team would deliver.

I carefully reviewed the data and contemplated how I would explain the potential financial loss to our board of directors and shareholders if we failed. In spite of the inherent risks, I was confident that we had both a capable team with a high level of technical and practical expertise and a clearly defined purpose to make this mission a success. So, I looked up at Steve and said, "Let's do it."

Once we had all our analyses completed and our plan finalized, we again gathered in the satellite control room as Steve's team redirected the satellite toward the moon's gravitational field. Several days later, the satellite began falling into the moon and was accelerating. As predicted, the satellite spun around the moon and exited the moon's gravity with increased inertia. However, it was traveling slower than expected and did not have enough velocity to make it into its intended geosynchronous position above Earth.

I turned to Steve and asked him, "Has our mission failed?" Steve replied, "No. We have a contingency plan. We could again use the satellite's positioning jets to navigate it into a second slingshot around the moon, which should get us to the required inertia." It was not clear if we would be making space history or experiencing another space failure. I only said, "Good luck."

Miraculously, the second slingshot was a success, and the satellite gained enough speed to reach its desired position. The downside was that it had only enough fuel left for 50 percent of its original life. However, with half of the insurance payout in pocket and a viable satellite to sell at a reduced price, we were still better off than if we'd taken the full insurance payout and abandoned the satellite. Not only that, but we'd successfully turned a negative into a positive.

MY CANCER EXPERIENCE was in some ways like this slingshot around the moon. The stakes were high, the science was evolving, and there was great uncertainty. Clearly, the risk of losing one's life is far more critical than losing a satellite, but there are parallels.

One significant parallel is the power of hope and purpose in the face of adversity. We took a big chance with that satellite, not only due to the financial risk, but also because we were attempting a new and complex maneuver. Yet in the end we chose to rely on the hope that we could avoid catastrophe and, with a collective purpose, turn this potential loss into a win. Clearly our success was mostly based on science. All the hope in the world was not going to reposition that satellite. Yet our hope and drive to succeed helped motivate us to strive for a positive outcome.

In the same way, cancer survival is for the most part dependent on science. The type of cancer one has, the stage of the disease, the quality of treatments, and how one responds to cancer and treatments are the biggest factors that will dictate how it will impact your life. However, many experts agree that hope plays a significant role in how you engage in your care and perhaps even how you respond to treatments. While the extent of that effect is sometimes unclear, many patients and leading health care professionals believe that hope is very important to the overall cancer experience. It certainly helped me.

Cancer was not the only challenge I have faced where hope and purpose played an important role. Like many, I had my share of adversity in my personal life and business career. Yet time and time again, hope and purpose helped me overcome these challenges. When cancer came into my life, I often found myself turning to these past experiences to help me manage all the challenges associated with my disease. I believe we all learn lessons throughout our lives that we can apply to our struggle with cancer. That being said, this disease can generate such uncertainty, fear, and confusion, we can sometimes forget to apply the tools and knowledge that helped us overcome challenges in the past.

Cancer is a mighty blow, especially since it seems to attack indiscriminately. I was reasonably healthy, ate well, drank modestly, and exercised regularly. Yet I faced two life-threatening cancers. I am not alone. Cancer routinely affects those who have no history of serious illness and have diligently followed the tenets of a healthful life. It's as if a roulette wheel has names in the slots, and a ball called "cancer" bounces randomly until it falls upon some unlucky soul.

How do patients deal with the seemingly random bad luck of a cancer diagnosis and all the questions and uncertainty surrounding chronic or terminal disease? How do they find the right doctor and treatments? How do they manage work responsibilities and the side effects of treatment? What about the ultimate question of survival? All this uncertainty and confusion can bring seemingly unbearable depression and despair. How do patients find and maintain the hope and purpose they need to carry on?

I wrote this book to address these very issues and try to provide guidance on how to manage the many difficult challenges associated with cancer. To this end, I share personal stories of how hope and purpose helped me overcome the many challenges I faced with my two life-threatening cancers and associated diseases. I also include stories from other patients who have been able to maintain hope in the face of depression, anxiety, and hopelessness and transform their cancer experience into an opportunity to find new purpose and fulfillment. These stories inspire and teach all of us that no matter how bad it looks, there is almost always a path to hope.

In addition, I have shared expert advice, opinion, and guidance from some of the world's top cancer specialists, all of whom believe in the power of hope and purpose.

Dr. William Nelson, the director of the Sidney Kimmel Comprehensive Cancer Center at Johns Hopkins, says, "Cancer can make you reflect to the point that it makes you depressed; or, it can change the way you hope for things. This opportunity to reflect can be a gift, if you use it correctly."

Chapter 1

I WAS FIFTY-THREE YEARS OLD when I accepted the position as CEO at Hughes Electronics in Los Angeles, California. It was 1992, and I'd just finished working for thirty-one years at IBM, a stretch that took me from an entry-level systems engineer fresh out of college to a role as one of IBM's top executives. I loved working for IBM. However, I was ready for a new challenge.

The transition to my new job and new life was all-consuming. When I first arrived at Hughes, I spent most of my time getting to know the management team and learning about the company. My assistant, Lilly, and I set up meetings from 7:30 a.m. until 6:30 p.m. After work, I'd schedule additional "informal" dinner meetings with the men and women who ran Hughes.

It was during one of those busy mornings that I got a call from the director of the health clinic at Yale University School of Medicine in New Haven, Connecticut, where I had received my annual physical exams before taking the job at Hughes. I assumed he was just checking in with me, making sure I had all my necessary medical records for my new life on the West Coast. I did, however, think it a bit odd that the director was calling me, as we'd never talked in the past. Sure enough, after engaging briefly in civilities, he said, "Mr. Armstrong, I am terribly sorry for having to make this call."

I replied, "I don't understand, what are you sorry about?" He said, "It appears we made a mistake. For the last two years your blood counts have been declining, and we missed it. You have a serious problem."

These words had a profound and disturbing effect on me. I knew how to handle business-related problems; I faced them every day. The solutions were reasonably straightforward: define the problem, lay out the alternatives, come up with the best plan, allocate the right resources, and implement with appropriate measurements and accountability. But I'd never faced a serious health problem. I'd had a couple of high school and college football injuries, but nothing life-threatening. When I damaged something, I got it fixed. The only serious consequences from those injuries were a little recovery time and perhaps some minor limitations.

When I asked why my blood counts were low and what it meant, the director paused and then replied, "We believe you have leukemia."

It's difficult to explain what it's like to hear you might have cancer. There's a moment of disbelief . . . Did I hear correctly? Did he say leukemia? I thought the "serious problem" he was referring to might be anemia or some other easily treatable health issue. Cancer was in an entirely different league. We were not just talking about some minor adjustments to my lifestyle. My life was on the line.

As I sat at my desk, listening to the director of the Yale clinic tell me I might have cancer, everything around me intensified. The office at Hughes I had inherited from the previous CEO was much larger than I needed, and at that moment, it seemed almost cavernous. Looking out of the enormous office windows on that clear spring morning, I could see the Pacific Ocean. The sky was deep azure, and the fierce rising sun was bringing with it another blazing California day. For someone who grew up in Detroit, where summers were short, and the weather often gray and cold this time of year, the view from that window made all that was happening seem that much more surreal.

As I stared out into that flawless dark blue sky, all I kept thinking was, if I had leukemia, where were my symptoms?

Then, an awareness swept over me. I did not have my usual seemingly boundless energy—there had been moments, recently, when I found myself feeling somewhat fatigued. I'd written this off as the stress of a new job and relocating, both of which had upset my life's routine, including my daily exercise program. Now it seemed as if there was something much more sinister at play.

How was I going to manage a cancer diagnosis? I'd only been in Los Angeles a couple of months and didn't know a single doctor or good friend I could call on for help. I'd also just started a very challenging job, and people were expecting me to be at my best. My schedule was full and only getting busier, and there were many sensitive and important issues to manage. All of this was going to require a lot of stamina. Once I'd finished meeting the team and getting up to speed at our corporate office, I would need to make site visits to manufacturing facilities and development labs all over the country. I'd also need to spend time with our marketing team and call on government clients in Washington.

In addition to my heavy workload, running a large public company like Hughes carries with it considerable obligations and visibility. Each of our 83,000 employees would be looking to me for direction and leadership. These first few months were critical. Shareholders and the press would be assessing how the "new CEO" performed. It was imperative that I project a strong and healthy image. This would be challenging, even if I wasn't fighting a life-threatening disease.

Of course, the bigger question was about survival. Could I beat leukemia, or would leukemia beat me? With my limited understanding of the disease and treatments, I had no way of knowing which outcome was likelier.

As all these thoughts raced through my head, my first response to the director was, "What do I do now?" He told me he'd already referred me to one of the nation's top leukemia specialists, Dr. Robert Peter Gale, at the Jonsson Comprehensive Cancer Center, University of California, Los Angeles (UCLA). He gave me Dr. Gale's cell phone number and then (as if to put extra emphasis on how serious this was) said, "I recommend you call Dr. Gale as soon as we hang up."

I put down the receiver and immediately dialed Dr. Gale's number. The phone only rang a few times before Dr. Gale answered. He was polite but didn't waste much time with pleasantries. He told me to come in first thing the next morning for tests. I had many questions to ask, but I figured those could wait until my appointment. We agreed on a time and said goodbye.

When I hung up, I was pretty sure I had cancer. Why else would the director of the Yale clinic call me personally and set up an appointment with one of the nation's leading leukemia specialists? Why would Dr. Gale insist that I come to see him the very next morning?

> " Gone are the days when a general oncologist could know everything. Even if it is just for an initial opinion to chart a course of treatment, you should see a specialist at a cancer center. "
>
> —DR. JULIE BRAHMER

I didn't know it at the time, but in spite of the missed diagnosis, I was lucky that Yale had a National Cancer Institute (NCI)–designated comprehensive cancer center (see Sources Cited, NCI-Designated Cancer Centers 2019). The US government created the NCI Cancer Centers Program as part of the National Cancer Act of 1971. The program identifies centers in the United States that meet rigorous standards for transdisciplinary, state-of-the-art research focused on developing new and better approaches to preventing, diagnosing, and treating cancer. You'll find the latest knowledge, technology, and cutting-edge cancer treatments at these centers. If the doctors at Yale didn't know how to best treat my disease, they'd know who to call. In my case, they sent me directly to Dr. Gale.

There are NCI-designated cancer centers located throughout the country, which I have listed in the Resources section at the end of this book. However, for some people it may not be easy or convenient to go to one of these centers for the full course of their treatment. In such cases, doctors recommend that patients at least try to get a consultation at one of these centers, so that NCI-designated experts can recommend a course of treatment that a local oncologist can follow.

> " These cancer centers can provide a roadmap that doctors back home can follow. Taking that one trip might change your course of treatment. "
>
> —DR. VERED STEARNS

With many questions, uncertainties, and concerns related to cancer spinning around my head, I did my best to calm down so that I could call my wife, Anne, at our house in Darien, Connecticut, and deliver the troubling news. It was still only a "potential diagnosis," and I wanted to make sure to convey this with hope and not resignation.

Anne was busy closing down our home and life back East so that she could join me in L.A. We talked a little about her progress on getting our affairs settled and when she might be coming to California, and then I broke the news. I told her about my call with the Yale clinic. I tried to be calm and not waver. I told her about the missed tests and the low blood counts. Next came the most difficult words in our conversation.

"They think it may be leukemia."

As expected, these words had a tremendous impact on Anne. She screamed, "Oh no, Mike, that's awful!" The path of our thirty-one years together had just taken a dramatic turn. Everything—the new job, the move, our future, our family, our life—looked completely different through the lens of a potential leukemia diagnosis.

After the initial shock had settled, we began talking it through. I told her the clinic had recommended Dr. Gale, an expert in leukemia, and that I would see him the following morning. This news seemed to comfort her a little. The understanding that we had a plan, even if it only extended to the next day, was at least something to hold on to. Like me, Anne could read the writing on the wall and was pretty sure I had leukemia. However, we both agreed to hold off speculating on severity, treatments, and possible outcomes until we knew more from Dr. Gale.

The call with Anne gave me some badly needed support. Even though she was three thousand miles away, I felt her by my side. We were facing this together and were prepared to deal with whatever was on the horizon, realistically and honestly, as we had done with the many other challenges we'd faced.

We decided it would not be appropriate to share this news among our family and friends until we knew more. There were too many unknowns to drag a lot of other people into this and have them worry unnecessarily. It was enough for now just to process that I might have cancer and to prepare for my appointment with Dr. Gale the following day. We did, however, plan to share this with Jack, my physician brother, as we needed his counseling and advice on treatment options. We also decided to tell two of our close friends in Connecticut. Anne wanted someone in Darien to confide in, so she didn't have to face this all alone.

My knowledge of cancer was fairly rudimentary at the time, but I did know that some forms of leukemia have a pretty good survival rate. On the downside, I also knew that cancers that go undetected for long periods of time can be more problematic.

One of the worst aspects of my diagnosis was that Anne and I were on opposite sides of the country. We talked about her coming out to L.A. sooner than originally planned but decided to wait until we knew more from Dr. Gale.

My afternoon at work was naturally filled with thoughts of cancer: Why me? What did I do to deserve this? I exercised regularly, was careful with my diet, and had regular checkups by good doctors. This is one of the more puzzling and troubling aspects of the disease. It often strikes randomly and mercilessly, and nobody really knows why. I had a very busy afternoon, which took some of my focus away from the crushing news I'd just received. Nevertheless, it's pretty hard to ignore a possible cancer diagnosis, and I struggled to stay focused and responsive during my many scheduled meetings.

I would have loved to talk to someone and air my concerns. However, that was impossible, as I had decided not to share this news until I had more information. I'd even held off telling my brother Jack or our friends in Connecticut until Anne and I had a firm diagnosis.

On the way home, I stopped at a French restaurant in my neighborhood, picked up something to eat, and headed back to the condo. Throughout dinner and into the evening, I mentally and emotionally wrestled with the internal terror of potentially being on a new path of life with an undefined and perhaps much shorter timeline. As I was pretty sure I had leukemia, most of my thoughts centered on severity, treatment options, and outcomes. Would I be able to continue work, and in what capacity? Would I need to be hospitalized? Of course, my biggest concern was survival. My cancer had gone undetected for a long time. Were my odds of beating this thing at least fifty-fifty, or worse?

After a restless night, I was up the following morning at 7 a.m. I tried my best to relax and enjoy breakfast, but it was hard not to keep thinking about the impending meeting with

Dr. Gale and its possible outcomes. I kept checking my watch, but the minutes seemed to creep by until it was finally time to head down the seventeen floors to the garage for the drive to UCLA.

Dr. Gale's office was much like any doctor's office, with a small waiting room out front. After signing in and a brief wait, a nurse showed me to an exam room. Soon the door opened, and a relatively young man appeared and introduced himself as Dr. Bob Gale. Without hesitation, he got right to the point. He told me he'd reviewed all of my records from the medical center in Connecticut and confirmed that my blood counts were very low and had been for a while. He would be able to tell me more once he had a clear diagnosis, which would require a sample of my bone marrow. It sounded like a surgical procedure, so I asked if he planned to "put me out." He said that wasn't necessary and told me he'd do the procedure in the exam room that very moment.

Dr. Gale asked me to lie down on the exam table and explained that he would first anesthetize the area and then insert a rather large needle into my hipbone. He cautioned that there would be some discomfort, but he would try to make it as quick and painless as possible. I prepared myself as best as I could, but with my low blood counts, the procedure proved to be too much, and I briefly fainted when Dr. Gale withdrew the needle. After I regained consciousness, he helped me sit up and told me to rest in the examination room until I felt strong enough to walk to my car. He said he'd call in a couple days with the lab results. After he left the room, I sat there for about ten minutes trying to get my energy back before beginning one of the slowest walks of my life back to my car.

Christine Hogdon was an avid runner who had competed in several half marathons. One day in November of 2014, while taking a shower after a twenty-mile bike ride, she found two lumps on her chest. She lived in Warrenton, Virginia and went to a small community hospital near her home to get things checked out. That was the start of a long dark journey into the world of cancer, according to Christine.

"The doctor told me the lumps were likely inflamed lymph nodes. He said, 'You're so young, you have no history of breast cancer in your family, you're fine. Come back in a couple months.' Even though I felt uneasy waiting, I trusted this doctor, this breast surgeon, who I was sure knew more than I did."

It wasn't until March, four months after that first visit, that Christine's doctor performed an ultrasound and told her that the lumps looked "suspicious." Instead of testing the lumps for cancer before surgery, he first removed them and then concluded they were cancerous. Christine later learned that this is "highly unorthodox."

This was not Christine's first experience with cancer. Her father had been diagnosed with a rare form of cancer in 2009 and died only three months later. The one thing she and her family always regretted was never having gotten a second opinion. She decided she wouldn't make the same mistake and made an appointment to see a highly recommended breast cancer specialist at an NCI-designated comprehensive cancer center.

"I was thirty-four years old with metastatic cancer, I was not messing around."

Chapter 2

BACK IN MY OFFICE at Hughes a few days after my appointment at UCLA, my assistant, Lilly, buzzed and said Dr. Gale was on the phone. My spine stiffened as I lifted the receiver. In his typical fashion, Dr. Gale did not waste time and got right to the point.

"Mr. Armstrong, the test results conclude that you have leukemia."

He went on to explain that I had hairy cell leukemia, which gets its name from the "hairy" appearance of the cancerous B cells when viewed under a microscope. He said that although it is not the most aggressive form of leukemia, my case was relatively serious because it had gone undetected for so long. He went on to explain that there were a number of Food and Drug Administration (FDA)–approved therapies that might work in my case.

However, there was also a new drug, called Pentostatin, which was especially effective with my type of cancer. He said that the drug was still being tested and was not available on the market, but there was a 100-patient clinical trial of Pentostatin that still had room for one participant, and he was sure he could get me in.

Dr. Gale carefully explained the risks associated with trials. However, he said Pentostatin had already been shown to be not only relatively safe but also very successful. I replied that if he thought that was the best course of action, it was good enough for me, and I asked him how and when we could start. He set me up with an appointment to begin my therapy, and we said goodbye.

As I hung up the phone, I was glad that we had come up with a solid plan for fighting my leukemia. However, I also had to face the reality that I had cancer and it could kill me. Outside of my office, the California sky was still blue, and my office was still too large for my needs. However, my inner world had drastically changed. I had moved from the land of those without cancer to the land of those with cancer, and it was terrifying.

Before that moment, there were two situations in my life in which I'd had to actually face the real possibility of dying. One of those happened in the early 1960s, when I was flying in a McDonald Douglas DC-3 from an IBM training session in Poughkeepsie, New York to my home to Indianapolis, Indiana. In the days before turbine engines were prolific, many commercial airplanes (like the DC-3) still used piston engines, which were much less reliable. Throughout my years at IBM, I flew on quite a few of these basic aircraft.

Including me, there were only eight passengers on the plane, all looking forward to the weekend at home. About thirty minutes into the flight, we suddenly lost altitude as the plane took a huge dip. We finally leveled out, but (as one might expect) there were some shrieks and commotion among the passengers who, like me, wanted to know what was going on.

A few minutes later, the co-pilot came into the main cabin and told us the right engine failed and they were unable to restart it. He said we'd be making an emergency landing at a nearby small airfield, only first we'd have to circle the airfield to burn off fuel. He then quickly returned to the cockpit.

Some of us began feverishly discussing the various possible outcomes of trying to land with only one engine. The consensus seemed to be that there were three possibilities: (1) we would land safely; (2) we would crash land and survive; or (3) we would crash land and not survive. This last scenario gave us all pause, and the conversations grew quieter and less frequent as each of us tried to cope with the reality that we might not survive the day.

Suddenly faced with what were possibly my last minutes on Earth, I thought about how random and unfair death can be, which is much the same way I feel about cancer. As we circled the airport, my thoughts gradually shifted from death and the various terrifying scenarios we faced to a kind of acceptance and hope in life. Yes, I could die in a fiery crash, but I also stood a good chance of surviving. Thus, with more hope than fear, I nervously waited as the plane finally descended and landed safely.

My second near-death experience also occurred on a flight home to Indianapolis. This time I was flying from Chicago, where I had started a new job as executive assistant to the IBM regional vice president. It was a Friday afternoon, and I took a cab from my midtown office to Midway Airport to catch a one-and-a-half-hour charter flight to the Indianapolis Airport. It was a small plane with one engine and six seats. I was the only passenger, so I was allowed to climb into the co-pilot's seat.

About twenty-five minutes into the flight, I smelled smoke in the cabin. The pilot and I stared at each other for a moment and then immediately looked behind us, where we saw an increasing amount of smoke coming from behind the rear cabin wall. The pilot quickly reached across me, pulled out a fire extinguisher, unlocked it, tested it, and handed it to me.

He said, "Mike, we have a fire back there. Take this and try to put it out. I will return to Midway as quickly as possible." Since we had just left the airport and were full of fuel, we were pretty much a flying bomb, which even the smallest fire could ignite.

Off came my seat belt, and I climbed back to the rear cabin wall where I saw a small door. I opened it, and even more smoke poured into the cabin. I couldn't see any fire, but I did my best to aim the extinguisher where the smoke was thickest. The pilot had opened the window beside him, as well as the one by the co-pilot's seat, and the cabin eventually cleared.

For the rest of our flight back to Midway I stayed next to the rear cabin wall, extinguisher in hand. I had never experienced a longer twenty-five minutes in my life. When we finally landed, I spent a very relieved night in Chicago, thankful to be alive.

In both of these scenarios, the possibility of death was relatively imminent. With cancer, I had much more time to think about it. I desperately wanted to call Anne and tell her that Dr. Gale had confirmed that I had leukemia and had outlined a treatment plan, but I had a very busy afternoon and didn't want to rush our call. I decided to wait until after work, when I would have time to consider the best way to break the news. I didn't want to seem depressed or present it as a death sentence. If I burdened her with "it may be over," I would evoke only grief and sadness.

As I worked through my busy afternoon, my thoughts shuttled back and forth between doubt and hope, anxiety and determination, fear and confidence. Especially troubling was the general ambiguity of the impending medical journey and fight for my life, as I had no clear sense of either a cause or a cure.

Once again, I tried to manage my emotional reaction to this news and examine the facts. Years of working as a senior executive had taught me this. If I let my mind wander down the rabbit holes of grief and despair, I could find myself lost in a wide range of scenarios that might not ever happen. The only things I knew for sure were: (1) I had a less aggressive form of leukemia, but it had gone unnoticed for a long time, so I had a serious fight on my hands; (2) the disease had lowered my blood counts, and chemotherapy would lower them even further, which meant I would be both tired and susceptible to diseases; (3) I would be participating for thirty days in a clinical trial that a leading cancer specialist believed was the best course of treatment for my type of cancer.

The treatment could fail, or it could work. These were both maybes, but neither of them was my current reality. I'd have plenty of time to address those "maybes" when they became "realities." However, in order to make the best decisions and take the best course of action, I needed to stay focused on what was definite and known and dismiss all speculation. I have experienced this kind of situation time and time again in my long career as a corporate executive, and I've learned that the best decisions always come from looking at facts, not fantasy.

In the 1980s, I was transferred to Paris to head up IBM's operations in Europe, Africa, and the Soviet Union. During that time, I learned that IBM's French mainframe software division was losing business to one of our French competitors. It seemed that as soon as we came out with a new mainframe computer software system, our competitor quickly responded with a product that was suspiciously similar to ours. After this had happened a number of times, we began to suspect that this company was somehow stealing our software designs and coding.

What made this problem particularly sensitive was that the French government owned a majority share of this competitor. If we accused our competitor of stealing software and didn't have the evidence to back it up, it could have significant political repercussions and could affect both our market interests in France and our reputation in Europe.

Before making a move, we first consulted with several US government officials. They agreed that we needed to confirm exactly how our competitor was gaining access to our software before we made any accusations. To this end, these officials recommended we purchase some powerful, "undetectable" cameras and install them in the ceiling of our IBM software development facility in Paris. Two weeks after installing the cameras, we discovered that two of our French IBM software engineers were copying coding sheets in the early morning hours, when the facility was officially closed.

We assumed that the French government had no idea of what was going on, and we also assumed that, like us, they'd prefer to keep this quiet. I arranged to meet privately with a high-ranking member of the French government, and I showed him the original IBM software code, the copied code, and a video of the IBM development men making the copies. The French official thanked me for bringing this to his attention, assured me that this kind of thing would never happen again, and the perpetrators were immediately and quietly removed from their positions.

Granted, when your life is in the balance, it's much harder to prevent emotions from clouding your judgment. Still, I did my best to stay relatively objective and examine only the hard facts regarding my cancer and my options. That being said, when you first learn you have cancer, there's a lot of information to process, and it's not always easy to separate fact from fiction.

Without question, the best source of information is your care team. Not only are they highly trained, but they also have direct up-to-date knowledge of the exact nature of your disease. I was lucky in that I had a physician who was both an expert on my particular type of cancer and also someone I trusted and felt comfortable talking to about my care.

> " When you hear that you have cancer, it's a big shock. You want to look up a lot of things, and you hear a lot of things from others. However, it's important to consider only high-quality opinions and reputable websites. You need to know your resources. "
>
> —DR. VERED STEARNS

After many years of doing business, making decisions, and concluding deals, I had a lot of experience assessing people's strengths and abilities. Dr. Gale impressed me as someone who was intelligent, competent, and friendly, but who did not linger or waste time. He had both my confidence and respect, and I felt very lucky to be under his care. What I especially liked about

Dr. Gale was that he didn't mess around. He gave me all the facts, and he gave them to me unfiltered and unadulterated. I personally prefer to hear news clearly and directly without a "spoonful of honey." He was both upbeat and realistic about my chances. He told me he was confident that this new chemotherapy treatment could beat my leukemia. I specifically noticed that he used the word *could* not *would*. He was honest, and I respected that.

There is really no gold standard for patient-doctor communication. Everyone has a different style, one that works best for them. For some patients, a warm and engaging bedside manner makes them feel comfortable and relaxed. Others, like me, prefer just getting the facts and don't need a lot of handholding. No matter how you like to communicate, the most important thing is that you feel comfortable asking your doctor questions and that he or she responds in a way that works for you.

> "Good cancer care is dependent on good communication between doctor and patient. You need to find a physician team that you're comfortable working with, that will not only provide the best treatment but also connect you with other treatment options. Make sure your medical team is doing what is best for you. If you don't feel comfortable or don't have productive communication with your doctor, you're likely not getting the most out of your care."
>
> —DR. VERED STEARNS

In addition to talking to your doctor, there is a lot of valuable information on the internet; however, you need to be selective about what you believe, as there's also a lot of misinformation.

I listed some reputable websites in the Resources section at the back of the book; you can also trust the websites of reputable medical institutions, such as Johns Hopkins, Yale, the

Mayo Clinic, MD Anderson, and others. There's also helpful information on the websites of disease-focused, not-for-profit patient-advocacy organizations. However, be cautious of these sites. You'll want to research the exact nature and purpose of any organization, to confirm that it is truly an independent, non-biased source. You should also look for the source (through footnotes or reference links) of any and all data you read on these sites and then check to confirm whether each source is legitimate. If information is not referenced by a dependable source, consider it suspicious until proven otherwise. The Society of Integrated Technology has a great page that provides useful advice on how to gauge the credibility of information found on the internet (see Sources Cited, SIO 2019).

The best data comes from peer-reviewed scientific studies published in reputable scientific journals. These studies are the gold standard for all medical treatments, drugs, and therapies. The world's top experts research and write these studies, and they adhere to rigid scientific principles to help ensure that the results are accurate and unbiased. Furthermore, independent experts meticulously review and scrutinize these studies before they're published and accepted as fact.

Whatever you find and wherever you find it (magazine, television, the internet, word of mouth, chat group, etc.), run it by your oncologist. If he or she finds reason to doubt the source, you should too.

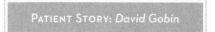

PATIENT STORY: *David Gobin*

David Gobin spent most of his life working as a police officer in a major East Coast city. In April of 2008, he was diagnosed with stage 2 non-small cell lung cancer, and his life changed dramatically.

The local oncologist who diagnosed him had a terrible bedside manner. "All he told me was, 'Go home. You've got three months to live. Go home.'" David says he had gone to a local oncologist because it was more convenient than driving an hour in traffic to the nearest major cancer center.

This local oncologist wanted to start David on chemotherapy and radiation, but he first wanted to take out David's entire afflicted lung. "I asked him, 'You want to take my lung out, where the cancer is? Why do I also need chemotherapy and radiation?' He was like, 'I'm God. I know.' That's the feeling I got. I thought he was a little condescending toward me. I said to myself, 'Hmm. I'm not having a lot of confidence here.'"

Not comfortable with his relationship with his local oncologist, David decided to make the hour-long drive to see an oncologist at an NCI-designated cancer center. "When I told my first oncologist that I was going to a cancer center for a second opinion, he said 'Oh, the Ivory Towers.' That's what he called it."

David says the way the doctor at the cancer center talked to him and treated him gave him much more confidence. "Her bedside manner was so great. Oh, my gosh, it was wonderful." David's new medical team enrolled him in a series of clinical trials that extended his initial three-month prognosis to more than a decade at the time this book was written. "All I can say is, if you don't like your doctor, find a doctor you do like."

The doctors at the cancer center told David there was no way to say how long he would live since none of them had a "crystal ball." "I loved that. They were honest but upbeat; they made me feel such relief." David says he'd like to go back to that first doctor and say, "Hello, still living!"

Chapter 3

As I stated earlier, I was very fortunate that Yale had an NCI-designated comprehensive cancer center and was able to refer me to Dr. Gale. He's not only one of the best leukemia specialists in the nation but also an avid researcher who was up-to-date on the latest developments in leukemia treatments and trials. In fact, Dr. Gale said my subtype of leukemia, hairy cell, was so rare that most general oncologists and even some specialists might not have correctly diagnosed it, much less enrolled me in a clinical trial specific to that disease.

> " Some of my patients wouldn't be alive except for the fact that they were willing to be part of a clinical trial that worked for them. The best person to talk to is your oncologist. You should ask 'What about clinical trials? What are my options?' "
>
> —DR. JULIE BRAHMER

A clinical trial is the process in which all drugs, therapies, and approaches to treating cancer are discovered, studied, and approved for general use. In this sense, clinical trials represent the front line of cancer research. These are exciting times, in that there are a lot of promising new therapies on the horizon. It can, however, take many years for these new drugs and treatments to be proven safe and effective for general use. Participating in clinical trials is like a journey into the future that enables early access to these new therapies. For some patients with advanced or difficult cancers and for whom all other options have failed, these trials may represent their only viable option for stopping the disease. However, like all pioneering voyages, there are risks, and one must understand the full implications of a clinical trial before considering enrolling.

Dr. Gale has spent a good deal of his career working with patients in clinical trials, and while he agrees that the future of cancer research depends on these trials, he also cautions that patients should clearly understand a clinical trial before signing on. The primary purpose of most trials of emerging therapies is not to "cure" the patients in the trial, but to learn more about a therapy, good or bad. In this sense, a clinical trial could potentially make you worse rather than better.

To clarify further, in order to gain FDA approval and be available for general public use, a drug must pass sequentially through "phases" of human trials that range from 0 through 3. A phase 0 trial examines how the body processes a new therapy and how the new therapy affects the body. These trials involve small doses and small groups, say ten to fifteen people.

Once a drug passes a phase 0 trial, it moves on to a phase 1 trial. This phase includes fifteen to thirty patients and gauges the safety of a drug by looking at dosage levels that produce the fewest side effects. A phase 2 trial looks at both safety and efficacy in a larger group of people (up to 100). Once a drug has successfully passed these phases, it must enter and pass a phase 3 trial before it is approved for general public use. Phase 3 trials typically include 100 or more patients and compare the new drug to an approved drug that is currently used to treat a specific disease. There is also a phase 4 trial, which rates the efficacy of new drugs already approved by the FDA. Phase 4 trials look more closely at side effects and can involve hundreds or thousands of patients. (see Sources Cited, NCCN, Phases of Clinical Trials 2019).

Dr. Gale said that only about 10 percent of phase 2 trials are successful, and phase 3 trials have a success rate of only about

50 percent. Not only that, since most phase 3 trials give only half the patients the new therapy (and the other half a placebo or a previously approved treatment), only about 25 percent of patients stand a chance of benefiting. Furthermore, "success" does not mean "cure." Sometimes it can merely mean the treatment has increased a patient's life by a relatively short amount of time, perhaps twelve to fourteen months.

> " People failing reasonable available therapies should consider clinical trials. However, they need to know clinical trials are done because we do not know whether a new drug or intervention is safe and effective. Patients should not assume a new drug or intervention used in a clinical trial is going to work and that they will benefit. In truth, the drug or intervention may not work and it is possible they may not benefit or even be harmed. Clinical trials are important because they offer hope when there may otherwise be none, because they advance science and medicine, and because they may help people in the future with the same problem. Therapies we use today were developed because people in the past were willing to participate in clinical trials. It is a noble deed. "
>
> —DR. ROBERT GALE

Once you look at all the facts, there's a lot to consider before you decide to enter a trial. Even if you're at the point where all other options have been exhausted and death is impending, you still need to give it careful consideration. Do you want to spend the rest of your remaining days driving back and forth to a medical center (and perhaps suffering some very unpleasant side effects) to gain only a possible short extension of your life? Or, do you want to spend your precious remaining moments with family and friends, enjoying these last few days, weeks, months doing what you want, surrounded by comfort and your favorite things and people? Dr. Gale said that just getting your blood tested at UCLA can take most of your day, given all the hassles with traffic, parking, and long wait times.

In my case, Dr. Gale assured me that Pentostatin, although not yet available to the general public, had already exhibited a high level of safety and efficacy, so the risk was relatively low. Furthermore, the treatment regime was easy to follow and would not upset my daily routine. He said that my other options at the time were having my spleen removed and taking a drug called Interferon. These options would have been much more involved and invasive. Also, they would have likely bought me only a short amount of time before my cancer returned.

> " You don't have to be in an oncologist's office to be matched up with a trial. There are a number of websites that are helpful. For example, the organization LUNGevity has a matching process that gives lung cancer patients a good insight into what trials are out there for their type of disease. "
>
> —DR. JULIE BRAHMER

All patients should be aware of clinical trials as a possible option if approved therapies fail. I list some useful information in the Resources section at the end of this book regarding clinical trials and where to find them.

Just make sure you have thoroughly examined all the risks and benefits as well as your specific needs, motivations, intentions, preferences, and expectations before signing up. The best place to inquire about trials is with your care team. The internet also has information about clinical trials for your type of cancer. Just be sure you're looking at vetted sites from reputable sources.

Dr. Nilo Azad had a thirty-eight-year-old patient with metastatic colorectal cancer. By the time he finally arrived at Johns Hopkins Hospital, all his former treatments had failed. "When I met him, I walked into the room and he was lying on the table. He couldn't even sit up, he was in so much pain. He was so weakened, he was barely eating. He said to me (which very few people say directly), 'I don't want to die.'"

Dr. Azad called the head of colorectal surgery at Johns Hopkins to see what they could do. The patient's cancer was concentrated in his pelvis and had not metastasized to any other parts of his body. They decided to perform a massive surgery, which took out all his pelvic organs. Sadly, within a month or two, his cancer recurred.

However, that couple of months bought him enough time to enroll in a new immunotherapy trial for a drug called a PD-1 inhibitor. This drug works best in patients with microsatellite instability—a genetic instability in tumors that creates a lot of mutations. Only about 3–5 percent of persons with colorectal cancer have this genetic trait; this patient was part of that small group.

He started that trial in 2014 and was still alive six years later, with no cancer. "He took an intravenous drug once every few weeks for a couple of years and is now off the therapy. The cancer's gone, and he's doing wonderfully. We're now at a point where we don't even know how often to scan him, because we don't know what to do in this circumstance."

Chapter 4

When I got back to my condo after work, the first thing I did was call Anne to let her know the test had come back positive for leukemia. I explained that Dr. Gale was enrolling me in a clinical trial that would begin immediately and last for thirty days and that he was confident it would be successful.

Throughout our life together, Anne and I always faced adversity with the same focus and commitment with which we faced opportunity. It would be no different with this cancer. We knew we had to stay positive and deal with this challenge head-on, with the shared hope that I would survive. We once again discussed whether she should come out and stay with me during my treatment, but we both knew that I'd be busy at work, and she'd be stuck in the condo with nothing to do. With all she had to handle back in Connecticut, wrapping up our former life, we decided it was best for her to stay there for the time being; if my condition got worse, she could always fly out. So we said goodbye, and I prepared myself for my thirty-day chemotherapy treatment regime.

I am left-handed, so Dr. Gale placed the intravenous line in my right arm. The chemotherapy pack attached to my belt in back with two loops and contained enough Pentostatin to last for the entire month of treatment. The pack was a soft, four-by-six-by-two-inch plastic rectangular pouch with a concealed thin plastic tube that went under my shirt and down my arm. When I took off my coat, only the chemotherapy pack was exposed, but not the tube—that's assuming I never rolled up my sleeves high enough to expose where the needle went into my arm.

I had to be especially careful that the needle stayed inserted in my arm and the line connected to the pack. Dr. Gale specifically told me that in order to have the best chance of success, the drugs had to flow continuously for the full thirty days of treatment. That meant I had to make sure I didn't pull it out accidently while sleeping at night. In addition, exercise of any kind, except walking, was out. There was too much risk of disconnecting the flow of chemotherapy and jeopardizing my chance of recovery. This was especially troubling for me, as exercise was an important daily therapy that helped me psychologically and physically manage the high-level pace and stress of work and life.

One of my first challenges was figuring out how I was going to explain to my colleagues at Hughes why I had a chemotherapy pack strapped to my waist and a tube in my arm, without telling them I had cancer and thus raising concern.

There are certain unique responsibilities and challenges associated with being the new CEO of a large public company. If word got out that I was battling cancer, it would send a confusing message to employees, customers, and shareholders. It would create uncertainty regarding both my ability to perform during treatment and my chances for survival. This would result in a loss of confidence and questioning of leadership that could have a negative effect on our sales and our market value. Therefore, it made sense to consider sharing the news publicly only if my treatment failed.

Of course, this decision was not mine alone to make. There were two very important entities I needed to consult with—the board of directors at Hughes and also the board at General Motors, which had a controlling share of Hughes. GM's CEO, Bob Stempel, was both supportive and sympathetic to my situation and agreed it was best to "wait and see." Similarly, each of the Hughes board members also expressed concern and support, and they agreed not to consider announcing anything until we knew the outcome of my treatment in thirty days.

The next item I needed to address was my stamina. As the new CEO, I had an incredibly busy schedule, which included extensive travel, meetings, and work-related social events. Chemotherapy was going to diminish my already low blood counts, which would make me even weaker. Thus, I would need to reduce my workload and cancel travel for the next thirty days. In addition to rearranging my schedule, my assistant Lilly would likely have to handle some sensitive incoming calls regarding my health status. Therefore, it was imperative that I tell her what I was going through and brief her on how to deal with any question that might arise.

I asked Lilly to come into my office and told her about my cancer diagnosis and treatment. She was visibly shocked to learn about my cancer, as she perceived me as someone with boundless energy and enthusiasm. She seemed especially upset when I told her that the cancer had advanced and I faced a very aggressive chemotherapy regime. We talked through my diagnosis and treatment, and I explained that she would need to reduce my schedule, cancel some appointments, and potentially field some sensitive calls regarding my health. Lilly provided a lot of emotional support and was a huge help during those difficult weeks. It was a tremendous relief to have someone in the office that I could talk to about what I was going through.

Before the cancer diagnosis, I had set up a number of meetings at various Hughes manufacturing facilities around the country, as well as trips to Washington to meet with defense officials. Now, with Lilly's help, I rescheduled those travel dates. I decided on an approach my daughters had taught me—tell the truth but not the entire truth. Lilly and I simply told my colleagues and customers that something had come up, and we had to postpone our meetings. Nobody asked any questions, and nobody seemed to mind.

The second thing we needed to address were my long workdays. Pre-cancer, I often worked ten to twelve hours a day, plus after-hours dinner meetings. However, with the chemotherapy and my dwindling stamina, I decided to shorten that to an eight-to-five workday and cut down on my after-hours work-related engagements. I also factored in some break time between meetings when I often enjoyed a Milky Way candy bar and/or a Coke to help boost my energy.

The only thing left to address was how I would explain the chemotherapy belt pack to my co-workers. Once again I decided to tell the truth but not the entire truth.

On my first day back at the office with my chemotherapy pack, I followed my routine of removing my jacket and hanging it in my office, which exposed the chemotherapy pack on my belt. At first, as expected, I got some strange looks from my colleagues. Before the questions came, I merely told them that for health reasons, my physician had asked me to wear this pack for the next thirty days. That seemed to do the trick, as nobody seemed to want to know more about it. After a week or so, everyone got used to it.

I suppose I was luckier than most in that I suffered very few side effects from the Pentostatin—there was no pain, itching, rash, nausea, or discomfort. As the weeks wore on, however, and my blood counts dropped due to the medication, I did start to feel more and more fatigue. It became increasingly difficult in the afternoons, when my energy and focus started to fade. My can of Coke and Milky Way bar routine helped, but there were times when I struggled to stay alert. Thankfully, the challenges associated with my new job offered some welcome distractions, which helped me manage my growing fatigue and the hovering reality that I was fighting a life-threatening disease.

Hard work has been a constant theme throughout my life, a theme that had been handed down through the generations. My father was the first person in our family to go to college. His parents were of limited means, so my father had to pay his own way. He spent his first two years living at home, working and

attending Wayne State University in Detroit. He then transferred to the University of Michigan, where he graduated with a
bachelor's degree in electrical engineering. My earliest recollec-
tion of Dad heading off to work was when he was employed at
one of the many defense plants that cropped up during the Second World War. I can vividly remember him leaving our house
very early in the morning and returning home late at night.

While a good part of my work ethic came from my family, it
was also a product of the era. The war was a time of hard work
and long hours in America. When I was going to public school
in Detroit in the 1940s, my classmates and I never took life,
grades, jobs, or opportunities for granted. The general rule was,
whatever you wanted, you had to earn it. This was not so much
a philosophy of life back then as it was a reality. There were no
free lunches and no short cuts. If you wanted promotions, rec-
ognition, or money—you had to compete, succeed, and deliver.

I started my first job when I was fifteen. Back then, I also
had a passion for horseback riding, and there was a ranch just
across the Detroit City line where I used to ride whenever I could
scrape together the money. For a middle-class boy from Detroit,
this was a rather expensive hobby, one that I would have never
asked my parents to finance. So, I applied for a summer job with
a contractor who specialized in building expansive "rolling"
landscapes for large luxury homes. The company used discarded
railroad ties in order to create the artificial "hills" on these prop-
erties. My job involved collecting discarded railroad ties from
the sides of railroad tracks and hauling them to the worksites.
The railroad company had no more use for these discarded ties
and was happy to have us take them away.

In order to get this job, given my young age, I needed to jump
through some hoops. First, I had to obtain a city work permit
and then qualify for a "provisional" commercial driver's license
so I could operate the truck the company used to collect the railroad ties. Both required a couple of letters of recommendation

and a number of interviews, but in the end, I got the license, the permit, and the job.

My co-workers and I would comb the railroad yards around Detroit, searching for railroad ties that were in good enough shape to reuse. Once we filled the truck, we'd deliver them to the worksites, where we'd hand-saw the ties to match the needs of each specific landscape design. Collecting and hauling those ties was a lot of work but also a lot of fun for a fifteen-year-old kid. It gave me both pride and a sense of being part of society.

Work plays a significant role in everyone's life, not just because it pays the bills, but because of how it defines us. We spend half of our waking days on the job; and for many, work provides significant meaning and purpose. When cancer enters your life, it is very disruptive. It can weaken your stamina, introduce doubt and uncertainty into your life, and even challenge your concept of life and death. In those difficult times, you need as much stability as you can muster to stay focused on treatments and survival and not be lost in despair and depression.

> " Cancer affects about 1-2 percent of the working
> population each year, which represents about
> 10-15 percent of an employer's annual health
> care costs. "
> **—SEE SOURCES CITED: WORKSTRIDE 2019**

Work can provide a strong structure for us to cling to while going through the ups and downs of this terrible disease. However, just as cancer disrupts our lives, it can also disrupt work. Treatments and appointments are difficult to manage and time-consuming, and they often require special compensation and understanding from our employers. There are also financial worries, as well as challenges regarding interactions with co-workers. To complicate this even further, our health insurance is often linked directly to our job. Successfully navigating these hurdles and finding a healthy balance between work and cancer is not only an enormous challenge but a necessity. After establishing a good relationship with your care team and a good treatment strategy, your next step should be to address how cancer will affect your work and how your work will affect your cancer. To this end, I've included information in the Resources section at the end of the book that can help you manage the delicate balance between work and cancer.

Chapter 5

As I APPROACHED the end of my chemotherapy treatment, the uncertainty and suspense regarding the outcome intensified. It was especially frustrating that there was no clear way of assessing whether I was winning or losing. With other types of illnesses, when a drug is doing its job, one starts to feel and look better. In my case, the Pentostatin was continuing to lower my blood counts. The longer I was taking it, the worse I felt, even if I was being "cured."

While a good night's sleep and a healthy breakfast boosted my morning energy, the afternoons became increasingly challenging, both physically and emotionally. Even more difficult were the evenings, when I was alone in my condo without the welcome distractions of work to keep my mind off of disease and uncertainty. I couldn't even enjoy an hour of post-work exercise or an evening drink.

After closing the door of my condo each night, I was alone with only my disease and treatment to occupy my thoughts. Was the chemotherapy killing my leukemia cells? Had it killed them all? Was I cured or just given a few more months or years to live? If I still had leukemia, would I need to continue the chemotherapy treatments? Were there other therapies? Adding to this was the greater isolation of being alone in L.A., with no family or close friends to talk with about what I was going through. I don't know what I would have done had it not been for my daily phone calls with Anne. This routine was something Anne and I had relied on throughout our relationship and marriage. They first started when fate sent Anne and me to different colleges after high school.

When I was young, Anne's family lived just down the street from my parents' house in Detroit. Anne and I met at a friend's party on the block, started dating in our early teens, and dated all the way through high school. We both planned to attend the University of Michigan, a Big Ten Conference school. The university had offered me a football scholarship and invited me and some other recruits to a game to get better acquainted with the team. We had seats right behind the players' bench, and it was the first time I seriously considered how big these guys were. Even in 1955, most linemen were 220–250 pounds.

It was clear to me that at 182 pounds, it would be difficult to compete with players so much bigger, and so I decided to attend Miami University of Ohio instead, where I was pretty sure I could also earn a scholarship (and did in my freshman year). Miami was in the Mid-American Football Conference, which also had a competitive football program, but the players were closer to my size. Anne, who was a year behind me in school, wanted to join me at Miami. However, her father was set on her attending Michigan, which meant we'd be apart during some very important years of our lives. As a result, I arranged to meet with him to see if I could change his mind.

Anne's father was a strong-willed, imposing man, and it was not without some trepidation that I met him in his living room one Sunday afternoon. I had known him for a long time, but since I was dating his oldest daughter, our relationship was somewhat awkward. (I know; I have three daughters.) In spite of this, he was a fair and honest man, so I hoped our conversation would go well.

Anne met me at the front door and took me into the living room where her dad was sitting in his large easy chair. I greeted him and shook his hand. It was a tense moment, and I knew it was up to me to start the conversation. I politely explained that I was confident I'd earn a football scholarship at Miami University and wanted to discuss the possibility of Anne joining me there instead of going to the University of Michigan.

Almost before I finished talking, he said, "Armstrong, the best I can figure out is that you'll end up selling popcorn in Tiger Stadium . . . end of discussion," and he left the room. For those unfamiliar with Detroit history, Tiger Stadium is where the Detroit Lions NFL football team played from 1938 to 1974. Thus, Anne's father was painting a rather bleak picture of my chances of succeeding in either football or college.

In those days, kids followed their parents' wishes. So, in spite of how much we wanted to be together, Anne went to the University of Michigan and I went to Miami University. Needless to say, we missed each other very much. We called each other frequently, and every chance I could, I'd go visit her.

I didn't have a car, so I'd hitchhike the 240 miles from Oxford, Ohio, to Ann Arbor, Michigan. I'd step onto the highway in Oxford around 11 a.m. on a Friday and stick out my thumb. After three to five rides, I'd usually roll into Ann Arbor just as the sun was setting. Anne lived in one of the university's women's dormitories, so I'd either bunk with a friend or rent a room. Sundays around 11 a.m., I was back on the highway, with my thumb out looking for a return trip to Oxford. I always dressed as a college student, with a sport coat and tie, which significantly increased my chances of getting rides.

When I was climbing the corporate ladder at IBM, we moved ten times. One week IBM would promote me to a new position in a new city, and the following week they'd expect me to be on the job. Anne would stay on where we'd been living until the kids finished school and she'd sold our house. I'd come home on weekends, but during the week we relied on daily calls to keep us connected. Now that I had been diagnosed with leukemia, I depended even more on that connection. She and I had been through a lot together, and this long history of love and support gave us the strength to face any challenge, including cancer.

When you have cancer, you need all the help you can get. In addition to support from friends and family, there are some great resources and great people available to help patients manage the wide array of cancer-related issues. One of the best places to look for support is through your care team. Many hospitals offer "nurse/patient navigators," who are trained specifically to help cancer patients with the difficult journey through their disease. Another great resource is "patient advocates" who, like nurse navigators, also help patients manage cancer's many challenges. Patient advocates generally operate independently of hospitals. However, your care team should be able to point you in the right direction. You can find information about various types of support in the Resources chapter.

> *Palliative care should start at the very beginning of treatment. It only makes sense to engage this team of specialists through the entire continuum of care to help with all the things that cancer and cancer treatments do to people.*
>
> **—DR. TOM SMITH**

An additional source of support that is often overlooked is your hospital's palliative care team. Many patients, and even some doctors, confuse palliative care with end-of-life care. The reality is that palliative care teams look at the full continuum of your care. Your oncologist often has their hands full just managing your cancer treatments and might not have the time or the expertise to adequately address other important issues associated with your disease. Johns Hopkins oncologist and palliative care specialist Dr. Tom Smith says his team not only ensures that patients are handling their treatments as well as possible but also addresses a wide variety of needs outside of medical care (depression, financial worries, transportation issues, work issues, etc.).

Patients should ask for palliative care as soon as they are diagnosed, according to Dr. Smith. He says palliative care not only provides improved quality of life, better symptoms management, and reduced anxiety and depression, it also can help patients live longer.

The American Society of Clinical Oncology strongly recommends providing palliative care along with regular oncology care for anyone with advanced cancer or significant symptoms from cancer (see Sources Cited, Ferrell et al. 2017). Dr. Smith says most large medical centers have palliative care teams, and many insurance companies cover the expense under something called "concurrent care," which provides for palliative care alongside oncology care.

PATIENT NAVIGATOR STORY: *Jill Mull*

As a patient navigator, Jill Mull works with breast cancer patients from the confusing and scary time of their diagnosis until they complete treatment, helping them facilitate the wide variety of challenges associated with their specific cancer experience. "The uncertainty of a cancer diagnosis brings a lot of fear and anxiety. You don't have a plan at that point, you don't know what's going to happen, you just think you're going to die," she says.

Talking to a professional who understands the landscape and who has practical advice and guidance can give cancer patients hope and a sense of stability as they develop and execute a care plan with their doctors. In this way, patient navigators serve as a helpful link between patients and the doctors, nurses, and other staff they will encounter throughout the treatment process.

Jill's passion for helping cancer patients is rooted in her own experience with breast cancer. She was diagnosed with HER2, triple-positive breast cancer, when she was only thirty-two years old. "My twins were four. I was feeling great, found a lump, and my whole world changed for the rest of my life—my career trajectory, my values, my everything."

Jill ended up having a bilateral mastectomy and a number of treatments, including chemotherapy and immunotherapy. Throughout it all, she was able to maintain hope due to the strong support she received from friends and family. "I had a community of support that was fantastic: my family, my husband, my parents, everybody. I was very lucky."

One of Jill's goals as a navigator is to try to provide that level of support. Generally, she joins new patients during their initial consult with the doctor, which is anywhere from sixty to ninety minutes. Jill tries to identify areas where she can make their life easier, such as finding transportation to care, managing side effects and other quality of life issues, balancing work obligations, and helping them with the Family and Medical Leave Act (which guarantees eligible employees time off for illness) (see Sources Cited, USGov. 2019). Jill also helps her patients deal with the financial difficulties of affording care by connecting them with resources that provide aid and even helping them with the often overwhelming amount of paperwork associated with the application process. "I'll do tons of paperwork until I get someone financial help."

Jill also leads support groups, which help connect cancer patients who might be going through similar experiences. "Peer-to-peer support is huge. I feel our support groups have been really helpful for people."

She says that fear and anxiety are crippling, but talking to other people who have similar disease issues can be a game changer. Everyone just wants to be normal, but the fear and anxiety cancer brings can make you feel like an outcast. Being able to talk to others is really healing. "As soon as the person sitting next to you, says, 'Oh, I had that treatment,' all of a sudden, it's normalized, and you don't feel that alone anymore."

Another important bit of advice Jill gives her patients is "Don't be afraid to call your doctor or treatment staff if you have a problem or questions, such as those involving side effects from your medication. There are often other medications available that are easier to manage. I tell my patients, 'Call! It's never a dumb call. We have a triage nurse who's sitting here waiting to hear your concerns. Please call us.'"

During her first chemotherapy, Jill had digestive issues commonly associated with chemotherapy that she tried to ignore. "Four days later, I'm in the emergency room at two in the morning. My entire family's panicked. I'm so sick. I'm buckling over in pain. We thought I needed to have my appendix removed, but it was something that could have been addressed with medication. Had I called my doctor, they would have prescribed me something and I would have been fine."

Jill also helps patients talk to their children about cancer, which can be very challenging. "When my son was four years old, I took off my wig to show him that I was bald, and he went away crying and screaming saying, 'Why didn't you ever tell me you were bald?' He thought I was bald his whole life. I said, 'No, honey, I'm bald because of the medicine.' He said, 'Why are you taking medicine that makes you bald?' That led to a conversation explaining how my hair loss was merely a side effect of my cancer treatment, and that this treatment would actually help get me better. I wish that a patient navigator had been available for me at that time for advice as to what to say to my kids.'"

Chapter 6

WHEN I AWOKE on the morning of the last day of my treatment and thought about what might happen in a few hours, my anxiety shifted to a sense of relief. I was glad the wait was over and ready to learn what the rest of my life was going to look like. I once again sat in front of my standard breakfast of coffee, juice, roll, and banana, continually checking and rechecking my watch until the time came to drive to the UCLA cancer center and find out who was winning this battle for life—me or leukemia.

In spite of traffic, I again arrived at the hospital early. I retraced my steps to Dr. Gale's office, checked in, and the receptionist showed me to an exam room. After a while, Dr. Gale came in with a warm handshake. We chatted a bit, and then he removed my chemotherapy pack and the tube in my arm, took a sample of my blood, and told me to wait until he checked to see if the Pentostatin had done its job.

It was a standard hospital exam room, but to me there was nothing standard about this moment. The 100th patient in a 100-patient leukemia clinical trial was going to learn whether this new chemotherapy treatment had worked. Not only would the answer impact many future leukemia patients, but I would either be cancer free or have a much more difficult fight on my hands—one that I might not win.

Throughout the previous month, work and life's other distractions had helped keep my mind off of potential outcomes. Given that this treatment regime was conveniently contained in a thirty-day envelope (that didn't even require a single hospital visit), I was able to push a good deal of my anxiety forward to the day when I would finish my treatment and learn the results. Now that day had come, and I felt as if I was waiting for the governor's pardon on death row. The seconds and minutes ticked away as I sat in that tiny cell-like examination room waiting for the knock on the door that would tell me what the rest of my life looked like and how much of it I had left.

Death is one of life's biggest mysteries. Luckily, we don't have to contemplate it much in our normal day-to-day lives. I first faced the reality of death when I was six years old. Back then, I spent many evenings lying on our living room carpet, listening to the latest World War II news on our large Zenith radio console. On Saturdays, I'd go to the Mercury Movie Theater around the corner from my house. In those days, before they ran the feature film, they played dramatic newsreels of savage battles raging across the globe. These scenes were both fantastic and terrifying, and they made it all seem very real to me. The war was not just on the radio and in the movies; it was part of our daily lives. Young men from our very neighborhood were off fighting in Europe and Asia, and those of us at home did our part rationing food and collecting scrap metal and rubber to be recycled for the war effort.

One of my weekly "WWII jobs" was crushing our used food cans behind our house and taking them to the edge of the road by the driveway, where a truck would pick them up. This was one of the ways I got to know my next-door neighbor Jim. Jim was in high school and a lot older than me. I'd see him when we were cutting grass, trimming hedges, carrying out garbage, or doing whatever chores our parents gave us. However, our most regular meetings were when we were out behind our homes crushing cans.

These meetings slowly developed into a kind of friendship. He was sixteen and I was six, so our interactions were not that complex. It wasn't really much more than a knowing nod or an occasional "How are you doing?" or "How many cans you got this week?" Over time, however, those casual encounters carried with them a kind of shared understanding and respect that we were the oldest boys in our families and had responsibilities.

After high school graduation, Jim joined the army and was soon shipped off to the war. Our weekly can-crushing sessions came to an end, but Jim always stayed in my thoughts and prayers. Every time I passed his house, I'd salute the red and white service flag with a blue star that hung in the front window and hope that he would come home safely. That flag was a daily reminder that my friend was far away fighting in a vicious world war.

One day, as I passed Jim's house, the service flag was gone. Instead, there was a gold star in the window. This sent a quiet but painful message to all in our neighborhood that Jim had been killed in action. I burst into tears and ran into my house, where my mother was waiting for me. I hugged her hard, thinking of my friend whom I'd never see again. This was very difficult for a six-year-old boy to comprehend.

My mother held me and said over and over, "We are so, so proud of Jim." When I finally calmed down and left her arms to go upstairs and change clothes, she said something that I have never forgotten. She said, "Mike, we will never give up hope."

> " My mother taught me that adversity is a natural part of life, and while we can't avoid life's difficult moments, we can try to view them through a larger lens, focused on a larger purpose. "
>
> —MIKE ARMSTRONG

For a six-year-old child, this first encounter with death was both confusing and terrifying. Yet these simple words from my mother seemed to ease my anxiety and sorrow over losing my friend Jim. It taught me that adversity is a natural part of life, and while we can't avoid life's difficult moments, we can try to view them through a larger lens, focused on a larger purpose.

These were not just words. My mother had faced her share of challenges. Her father had lost his job and all his savings in the Great Depression. He had a family to feed, so he went door-to-door looking for work. He finally landed a job with the U.S. Postal Service and stayed there until he retired. One of my mother's biggest dreams was to go to college. She wanted to contribute to and compete in society. However, given the times and the limited financial resources of her family, she never got the chance.

Everyone faces challenges in life; they are inevitable. However, it's not just about *what* happens or *why* . . . it's *how* we handle it that counts.

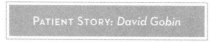

PATIENT STORY: *David Gobin*

One thing David Gobin likes to tell other cancer patients is, "Never give up hope."

"It doesn't matter how sick you feel. There will be days you feel good and days you don't. You can go in the corner and give up and die. Or, you can stand in the middle of the floor and say 'Come on—You want a piece of me? Come get me!' And that's what I decided to do. But I'm not saying it wasn't hard."

David's doctors, the internet, and everyone else told him that he'd only live a few months with his type of cancer. Yet at the time this book was written, he'd survived more than a decade. Granted, he is one of the lucky ones, but he still thinks that there should be more positive messages out there, especially in light of all the breakthroughs in cancer treatment that are happening daily.

"When I first got diagnosed, people would tell me how their aunt, uncle, sister, or brother died from cancer, and I'm like 'My God, don't you people have any stories of people who lived?' I need to know that people lived. People need to know that, they need hope. Don't take my hope away. All I ever wanted was hope."

Chapter 7

AFTER WHAT SEEMED like an eternity, Dr. Gale finally returned from the lab with my test results. He was smiling as he stepped through the door and, in his customary fashion, got right to the point. "Mike, your leukemia is gone. The chemotherapy did its job. It worked."

Words can't explain how happy I was to hear those words. Just as quickly as cancer had suddenly and unexpectedly entered my life, it was gone. In its wake, it had taught me how fragile and precious life was, and I was looking forward to returning with confidence to my life as husband, father, and grandfather and to my new job at Hughes.

Of course, I was not out of the woods yet. Dr. Gale explained that the chemotherapy had killed not only the cancer but also a good number of my blood cells, which we now had to rebuild. He told me it would take a couple of months and daily shots to rebuild my immune system. He handed me a box containing some vials and needles and showed me how to inject myself in the thigh. We shook hands, and I headed out of his office, cancer free.

On the drive from the hospital to Hughes, it felt as though I was starting a brand-new life. After a month of dangling at the end of a rope, chemotherapy had cut the hangman's noose. The huge smile on my face must have bewildered some of my fellow motorists in L.A.'s impossible stop-and-go traffic. With all this excitement and gratitude racing through my thoughts, I experienced a strong desire to do something to pay the world back for my good fortune. However, at that time I had no idea what that might be.

When I got to my office I picked up the phone, called Anne, and almost yelled, "The leukemia is gone!" She screamed with joy, started crying, and we repeatedly expressed our love and gratitude that I was back on the road to a healthy life. It was one of the happiest and most wonderful moments in our marriage. We had just made it over our toughest hurdle to date. For two people who had been through so much together, nothing was more valuable or precious than knowing we had more years to enjoy.

Facing mortality also made us realize how much we needed each other's company. As a result, we concluded that whatever work she was doing closing up the house in Connecticut was not as important as our being together. We decided she should join me in L.A. as soon as possible. We were beginning a new chapter in life and wanted to enjoy it together.

We hung up with the promise to talk later in the evening. I spent the rest of my day at work with a smiling confidence. My team might not have fully understood my newfound exuberance, but they seemed to enjoy it as much as I did. Lilly— the only one of my co-workers who really knew what I'd been through—was ecstatic that I was both cancer free and on the road to health again.

> "I experienced a strong desire to do something to pay the world back for my good fortune. However, at that time I had no idea what that might be."
> —MIKE ARMSTRONG

Back at the condo that evening, as I drifted off to sleep, I thought of all the wonderful years that lay ahead. My life, which had been cloudy and uncertain for the past thirty days, was now clear and bright. With all of these positive thoughts racing through my head, I had one of my best sleeps since I'd arrived in California—that is, until I woke up around midnight drenched in sweat.

Confused, achy, hot, and nauseous, I dragged myself out of bed, grabbed a thermometer from the bathroom cabinet, and took my temperature. It was 103 degrees! My first thought was that I'd caught the flu or eaten some bad food, and then it dawned on me that it was likely a side effect of my cancer treatment. After all, my immune system was all but nonexistent, thanks to a month of aggressive chemotherapy.

Dr. Gale had told me to use his cell phone number if I had any serious side effects from my treatment. I figured that a 103-degree temperature qualified, so in spite of the late hour, I called him. He picked up the phone after only two rings. I apologized for the late call and told him what was going on. He told me that I might have a blood infection and it was imperative I go to the hospital immediately.

All the joy I had been feeling evaporated in a rush of panic and fear. I told Dr. Gale that I didn't feel well enough to drive and asked him to send an ambulance. To my surprise and shock, he said, "Mike, that's not possible. Don't you know about the riots?" I had missed the evening news, so I asked, "What riots?" Dr. Gale explained that people in the city were rioting over the verdict on the Rodney King beatings. Every emergency vehicle in the city was engaged in restoring order, putting out fires, and rescuing people. In addition, taxis were either not operating or impossible to get because of the general chaos in the streets. The only way to get to the UCLA cancer center was to drive myself. He suggested I leave as soon as possible, before the riots got worse. There was no other option. Time was of the essence.

I gathered my car keys and whatever I thought I might need at the hospital. My primary focus was figuring out how I would navigate the riots and get to the hospital both quickly and safely.

However, I also felt frustrated and even a bit angry. Cancer had just put me through one of the most difficult and challenging months of my life. I had done all that was expected of me. I suffered through the exhaustion and discomfort of chemotherapy and managed to keep my work and life together. Now I was suffering from another life-threatening condition that was directly related to the very treatment that had saved my life.

While this seemed terribly unfair, the more I learned about cancer, the more I realized that many cancer patients face a similar rocky road, strewn with associated disease, cancer recurrence, and debilitating side effects, and yet they somehow manage to overcome these seemingly insurmountable odds.

PATIENT STORY: *Christine Hogdon*

A PET scan had shown some spots on Christine's thyroid and lung, so her oncologist ordered biopsies. The thyroid biopsy, while a little painful, went as planned. However, as the doctors were performing the biopsy on Christine's lung, it collapsed and would not reinflate.

"It was horrible. It was really painful. They had to place a chest tube to provide oxygen because without it, I felt like I was drowning. Even though just one of my lungs had collapsed, I couldn't breathe," Christine says. It took a week before her lung reinflated and she was able to begin her treatment regimen. The NCI-designated comprehensive cancer center was an hour's drive from her home, but she says it was well worth it: "I started all my treatments in May, and I finished chemo around Labor Day."

Christine lost all her hair due to her treatments, even her eyebrows and eye lashes. She was able to cover her thinning hair with a bandana but had not mastered the art of fake eyebrows or eyelashes. "My brother came to visit, and he said, 'You look weird. What's wrong with you? You really look weird.' I replied, 'I have no eyebrows, I have no eyelashes, thank you for noticing.'"

After four grueling months of weekly chemotherapy, Christine's road to recovery did not get any easier. "I decided to have my thyroid and the tumors in my breast removed at the same time so that I would only have to endure one surgery. I woke up with this huge gash across my neck where they had taken out the thyroid. A few weeks later, I developed a seroma under my arm, which is a painful pocket of lymphatic fluid that can develop after having lymph nodes removed."

They drained it several times, but it got infected, so she was given antibiotics. The antibiotics wiped out all her good bacteria, and she ended up with a Clostridium difficile (C. diff) infection, which is pretty dangerous. "I dropped down to about 100 pounds. I was so skinny. Everybody thought I was sick from cancer, but I told them, 'It's not even cancer, it's a stupid bacterial infection.' It just felt like more bad news, more bad news."

When she was recovering from the C. diff infection, Christine noticed that she kept biting her tongue. When she took a closer look in a mirror, she saw that her tongue was completely atrophied on one side and paralyzed. Her nurse recommended she go straight to the hospital, because she might be having a stroke. "My doctors thought I had a brain tumor. They did a spinal tap, a magnetic resonance image (MRI) of my brain, and a number of other tests, but in the end, they had no idea what caused it."

Christine believes that the paralysis was a permanent side effect of the chemotherapy. "My tongue was doing weird things throughout the chemo. I could feel sometimes it would go numb all of a sudden, and I remember thinking, 'That's weird.'"

To manage her disease means that Christine must get regular transfusions of targeted therapeutic antibody therapy every three weeks. For that she has a permanent port installed in her chest. "Once you're stage 4, the horse is out of the barn, so to speak." She says metastatic patients never get to downgrade and can never be cured, only managed. "We're basically keeping my cancer at bay with a combination of drugs."

If she's not showing any signs of cancer, doctors say she has "no evidence of disease," or NED. "Some patients say 'I'm dancing with NED,' or 'We're still flirting with NED.' You never know when it could come back. I could progress at any time, but we are prepared for that."

Christine says she is lucky in that she has been able to remain positive despite all that she has been through. "It's all about how you look at it; some people have it worse than I do. When I hear people complaining about traffic and other meaningless stuff, I'm like, 'Really? Come on guys!' That's one thing cancer does for you: it really puts things in perspective."

Christine doesn't think far ahead any more. She just tries to appreciate the time she has now. "When people say, 'What are you going to be doing next year,' I think, 'I might not be here next year.' I just don't know. Cancer helps you understand and respect that you never really have control of anything."

Chapter 8

I TOOK THE ELEVATOR down to the parking garage and got into my car. The 103-degree temperature not only had me sweating and exhausted, it also made it very difficult to sustain the focus and physical capabilities that I needed to successfully navigate through a rioting city. I had little or no experience with riots, but it seemed sensible that rioters would probably be lurking on the side streets to avoid being seen by the police, so I decided to stay on larger, busier roads whenever possible.

I wasn't worried about negotiating the upscale neighborhood of El Segundo, where I lived, or driving on Highway 405. What concerned me was that I would have to exit 405 and drive through the inner city to reach the UCLA cancer center. Essentially, I'd be driving through an area where the rioting could be intense. This was long before cars had GPS, and being new to the city, I didn't know any "safer" route. I didn't even have a map of Los Angeles in the car. Clearly, there was no other option. I'd simply have to face the inner city and whatever was going on there. If there was a confrontation, I'd just have to deal with it. With this rather simple plan, I pulled out of the condominium garage.

As expected, the streets were quiet in my immediate neighborhood. No signs of rioting. Regardless, I tried to maintain a heightened awareness of everything around me, which seemed only to push my fever higher; I was literally sweating through my clothes. Pulling onto 405, I noticed that the highway was eerily void of L.A.'s iconic traffic. Obviously, anyone with any sense was safe at home. The vehicles I did encounter were mostly police cars, fire trucks, and ambulances. They were all moving at an aggressive pace, but because there was very little civilian traffic, they had their sirens off, which only made things seem that much more surreal.

The section of 405 connecting El Segundo to the inner city often dips below street level, so I couldn't always gauge the full intensity of the rioting. However, I saw that the upper floors of several buildings were burning and could only imagine the chaos that was likely happening on the street. I gazed at my watch and estimated that in roughly fifteen minutes I'd have to exit the highway and possibly drive through all this madness. My condition was getting worse, and I had no idea how and if I was going to survive. Even if I were healthy, and clearly I was not, this would be a perilous journey.

Of course, I had little choice but to go on. If the gangs running wild in the streets didn't get me, the blood infection would. Exiting the freeway, my strength began to leave me. My fever was at a boiling point, my vision was blurred, and I felt both dizzy and nauseous. Unable to drive any farther, I pulled over to the curb, literally struggling just to stay conscious. However, passing out in downtown rioting L.A. was not an option.

The only time in my life when I had to deal with "gangs" was during my childhood back in Detroit. My family moved to another part of the city, and I needed to change to a new elementary school, one that served two very different neighborhoods: our residential community to the south and the "projects" to the north (a complex of low-cost housing units). There was a prowling gang of elementary-school-aged kids from the projects that regularly beat up the residential kids, especially new kids like me.

Whenever I encountered this group, they'd surround me and shout, shove, punch, and hurl insults. Eventually, one of the kids would challenge me to a fight. The rest of the group would keep me inside their circle so I couldn't escape.

Coming home pretty battered after my third gang encounter, my mom had seen enough and came up to my room. She sat down next to me on the bed, where I was nursing head wounds from pounding fists and leg bruises from kicks. She looked me over lovingly and gave me another strong dose of her positive philosophy.

"Mike, you must win these fights if you want them to stop. You just have to be tough enough to never give up, and you will win." With a big hug and a pat on the shoulder she walked out of the room, leaving me totally determined not to let her down.

> " My mother taught me how to look for hope and purpose throughout life, no matter what I was facing or how bad things were. "
> —MIKE ARMSTRONG

Just as she had done when my neighbor and friend Jim died in the war, my mother gave me something positive to focus on in the face of adversity. Instead of accepting things as they were, she encouraged me to hope and strive for a better outcome. I might succeed or I might fail, but at least I would be trying to make things better.

Up to that point, my strategy for dealing with the gang was to avoid them whenever possible. When they did find me, I'd weather the hits, kicks, insults, and punches until I could escape, and then I'd run as fast as I could all the way home. Now I had a new strategy. The next time I encountered those boys, I'd face them, not back down, and do whatever necessary to stop them from ever bothering me again.

Several days after that fateful talk with Mom, I once again encountered the gang while walking home from school. Instead of running away, I walked to a nearby empty lot and waited. There were about six of them, and they quickly surrounded me while shouting and taunting. Among them were some familiar faces and some new kids I had not seen before. After they finished with the insults-punches-and-kicks phase of the attack, one of them stepped forward to fight me.

I knew the routine all too well. Only this time, instead of just cowering and looking for a way to escape, I charged my attacker and met him head-on with my fists flying. My left shoulder hit him squarely on the chest and he went down backward with me on top of him. After I landed many solid punches, I got up and he stayed down. The gang closed in around me, but nobody said a single word and nobody stepped up to challenge me. I turned around and walked home. I never had any problems with those guys again.

A small group of eight- to ten-year-old kids is clearly not the same thing as a rioting L.A. However, there was one similarity. I had to focus on a positive outcome. I could not just give up. I had to make it to the hospital. I had to survive.

Struggling to stay conscious, I rolled down the car window, took a deep breath and managed to summon enough energy to pull away from the curb. I only hoped that I could remember how to get to the UCLA cancer center. There were a couple of key turns I had to make to navigate this area of L.A. The last thing I needed, on top of everything else, was to get lost.

Through my fever, confusion, dizziness, and the stress, I ignored whatever was going on around me and focused all the energy I had on trying to keep the car on the road. With this simple strategy, I somehow miraculously found my way without incident. When I finally saw the glow of the lights of the hospital through my dripping sweat, it was like a beacon of salvation, which brought me tremendous happiness and relief.

However, I wasn't quite there yet, I still had to make it from the parking lot to the main entrance. Throughout the drive to the hospital, the need to focus and my desire to make it safely had given me some temporary resilience. However, I now felt the full intensity of my illness. It required all the strength I could muster to swing my feet to the pavement and climb out of my car. Four or five steps into my walk, I got dizzy and had to grab the side of a parked car to prevent myself from falling. After a few minutes of deep breathing, I regained some strength and continued my slow, agonizing, wobbly journey to the hospital entrance.

Inside the UCLA cancer center, I had one last challenge—the long hallway that led to the admissions desk. I was literally on the verge of passing out with each step. When I finally made it to the end of the hall, an attendant with a wheelchair suddenly appeared. For the first time since I'd woken up sweating in my condo with a fever of 103 degrees, I sat down, relaxed, and let someone else take over. I couldn't believe I'd actually made it.

Chapter 9

THE ATTENDANT TOOK ME to an isolation room in the intensive care unit (ICU), which would be my home until either I or my infection was gone. After running a few tests, a nurse explained that, given that I likely had a blood infection and also a weak immune system, they were putting me in an antiseptically "clean room." She said that aside from Dr. Gale, the attending physician, and a couple of nurses, the door would remain closed to visitors. Not even my wife was allowed inside.

The nurse pointed to a small TV on the wall and a bedside telephone and told me that these would be my only contact with the outside world. With my isolation thus defined, the nurse gave me my first shot of antibiotics and left a sleeping pill on the bed stand. It was almost 2 a.m., and I was exhausted. I skipped the sleeping pill and fell fast asleep.

The next morning, I assessed what would be my new home for an undefined period of time. The walls were bright white, the floor spotless, and the chair had neither fabric nor cushions. The one window was crystal clean, and even the ceiling looked "sanitized." This was going to be a sterile and lonely stay.

Soon the door opened and Dr. Gale came in. His "Good morning Mike" and handshake were significantly more reserved than on the previous day when I'd visited his office and learned that my leukemia was in remission. He asked me how I was feeling. I told him I'd been doing great until this infection hit me. He smiled and then said rather matter-of-factly that I had a bloodstream infection and with my weakened immune system, it was spreading relatively unchecked. To treat it, they had given me a very powerful antibiotic. He assured me that we could beat this infection just as we'd beaten the leukemia, and then he left.

Alone in that stark isolation room, I struggled to understand what had transpired. I'd spent a difficult month battling and overcoming a dangerous life-threatening disease only to be thrown from that frying pan into a fire that burned with a much higher intensity and a shorter timeline. To make things even worse, I was also now effectively isolated from my wife, my work, and all that I loved about life.

The only other time I'd been confined to a hospital room was when I dislocated my right shoulder playing football in college. Like my blood infection, that shoulder injury also threatened to jeopardize my future, but in a different way. Surgical techniques were less developed in the 1950s than they are now, and my surgeon did his best to fix my shoulder with a tuck in the ligaments and a large steel staple affixed to the shoulder to hold the ligaments in place. The good news was that my shoulder still functioned pretty well, although the procedure had shortened my arm a bit and limited my rotation by 15 percent. The bad news was that my football days were over, and so was my scholarship. That same month, the company where my father worked went bankrupt, and he lost his job. With no scholarship and a challenging financial situation at home, I had no choice but to drop out of college.

At that point, my life could have gone in a number of different directions. However, I didn't lose hope in the possibility of graduating and came up with a plan to finish college. In spite of the recession that swept the country in the mid-1950s, I found a job working six nights a week at a flour mill on the Detroit River, loading 100- and 140-pound flour bags into boxcars.

The flour bags would come down a chute from the floor above. I would catch each bag head-high off the chute, tilt it onto my healthy shoulder, walk down the boxcar and stack the bags in rows, six to eight bags high. When the boxcar was full, I'd take the loading document to the supervisor and get my next boxcar assignment.

This exhausting routine, eight to twelve hours a night, six nights a week, got a little old at times. It was hardest when I was working the boxcar alone, which happened frequently, since I always signed up for overtime. This extra work added a much-needed additional five cents an hour, but I often didn't get home until two or three in the morning. As a result, I didn't have much of a social life.

A year after losing his job, my dad started a manufacturing representative business. With my family back on the path to solid financial footing and with the money I'd saved loading boxcars, I was able to return to Miami University. Back when I had first enrolled in the school, there were two primary goals: get an education and play football. Now I had only one goal: achieve an academic record that would enable me to find the best job opportunities.

After graduation, I landed a position selling and installing data-processing equipment for the IBM Data Processing Division in Indianapolis, Indiana, and I stayed with the company for thirty-one years.

Those kinds of lessons reminded me time and time again that no matter how bad it gets, hope and purpose can get you through almost anything. No matter how depressing it was in my isolation ICU room or how sick I felt, I desperately needed to maintain hope. The doctors would take care of the rest. That being said, finding hope is not always easy. Many strong individuals find it difficult to stay positive in the face of cancer. However, in the absence of hope, there's only despair and depression, which can make the already difficult challenges associated with cancer almost unbearable.

For many years, the intersection of hope and cancer has gotten little attention. Most hospitals and physicians are primarily focused on fighting the disease. Nevertheless, oncologists, clinicians, and even some hospitals are beginning to realize the importance of hope and incorporating it into their cancer care.

One of these clinicians is Anna Ferguson—a career oncology nurse and researcher who recently founded a program called Hope Matters to address the role hope plays in cancer. Anna says her life's work has shown her time and time again how important hope is in the struggle against cancer. To illustrate this, her team conducted hope enhancement workshops with stage 4 cancer patients and oncologists to look at what hope means to patients and to develop strategies to better manage hope. The workshops asked patients and clinicians a variety of questions about the role hope was playing in their cancer. The results clearly showed how hope is intertwined throughout the entire fabric of the cancer experience.

> " Humanity can be lost in medicine. A discussion about hope, specifically what a patient hopes for on a given day or from a given therapy, can be a portal to help bring that humanity back to medicine. "
>
> —NURSE-RESEARCHER ANNA FERGUSON

Anna said one of the most telling moments in the workshop was when both a patient and an oncologist gave her the same answer when asked to define hope. They both said that hope was the reason they were still here. For the oncologist, it was the reason he came to work every day, and for the patient it was what kept her engaged in her treatments and fighting to stay alive.

"Hope is where we connect as humans. It's no longer 'I am the well one over here and you are the sick one over there. You are in that funny gown and I am in my normal clothes.' Hope is where we meet; it is what we have in common," says Anna.

According to Anna, the purpose of her work is not only to create a culture shift and elevate this subject but also to educate clinicians and patients about the role and importance of hope and to develop tools for discussing and managing hope. She says someone once told her that if a hopeful attitude were a drug, the FDA would have approved it by now, and we'd be giving it to everyone twice a day.

NURSE STORY: *Anna Ferguson*

Anna Ferguson, career oncology nurse and researcher, says the importance of hope in cancer care became especially clear to her in 2008, when she was working to help connect a cancer patient with a clinical trial.

"It was one of those suboptimal patient-physician interactions," says Anna. Typically, the patient meets with the physician, and then Anna helps the patient fill out the necessary paperwork. This patient had a particularly difficult and debilitating cancer that was not responding to therapies. "The patient was very sick and very sad, and the family was sad; this trial in some ways represented their only hope." Anna says that the physician she was working with at the time was not responding to the emotion in the room or connecting well with the patient or his family. "The physician was kind of looking down, and I was watching and sort of knowing this wasn't going the right way. It wasn't working."

The physician left and the patient signed the paperwork. However, the patient failed to show up when the time came to start the trial. This was especially odd because this patient was well versed regarding the science behind the trial and had initially been motivated and enthusiastic to join.

Anna had a bad feeling. She knew the patient's medical condition was fragile and thought the patient might have died. She tried to call, but got no response for two weeks, until one day the spouse finally answered the phone. The caller ID must have shown on the phone, because the patient's spouse started yelling even before Anna had a chance to introduce herself.

"This very distressed and frustrated spouse kept yelling at me, 'What? What? What? What do you want?' And I knew, I knew the whole thing. It was a life-changing, soul-changing, career-changing moment."

Over her many years working with cancer patients, Anna has taken part in a lot of difficult phone calls. However, this call was particularly hard. "The patient's spouse just kept screaming, 'You left us no hope, how could we come back there? No hope! You left us no hope!' That call haunts me to this very day."

The only thing worse than so callously failing another person is not knowing exactly what you can do to prevent another failure the next time, according to Anna. She says it was not her best day working with a patient, but it was also not her worst day.

The patient's spouse told Anna that other hospitals and doctors had expressed similar opinions about how advanced the cancer was and how poor the chances were for survival. However, they at least left some hope.

This experience made Anna totally reexamine the role hope plays in cancer diagnoses and treatments. Anna says clinicians often do not know how to help patients find hope, especially when the prognosis is bad. They are reluctant to provide false hope and are equally adverse to taking away hope. Yet her many years working as a cancer clinician have taught her that hope is essential to the patient experience.

"Hope adds quality of life both to the physician and to the patient. It is the undercurrent of all we do in oncology. The same is true of all medicine. Hope transcends age, gender, health, status, and treatments."

She added that perhaps one of the potential reasons why hope has been overlooked in the treatment regime is because it is difficult to measure and quantify.

"Hope is defined differently for everyone in the setting of bad news," she says. "It was the same in the past when we tried to quantify pain. Today we have pain scales that make it easier for physicians to gauge how much pain a person is experiencing. Can we do the same with hope?"

Chapter 10

I HADN'T CALLED ANNE when I was admitted the night before, so I phoned our house in Darien and told her all I'd been through since I had woken up in my condo sweating and dizzy with a temperature of 103 degrees. She was understandably very concerned and wanted to get on the next flight to L.A. I told her that I'd love to have her by my side, but I was in an isolation room, and the doctors wouldn't let anyone in the room except hospital staff. We agreed to wait until I was out of the ICU, and I promised to call again in the evening.

The rest of the day seemed to drag on, as there really wasn't much to do in that lonely ICU room. Finally, the attending physician came in to check my blood. Unfortunately, there wasn't any improvement. Sensing my disappointment, he told me not to worry, that the antibiotics should work.

When I woke up the next day, my fever and nausea were gone, and I was feeling markedly stronger. Surely, the antibiotics must be working. With a positive sense of anticipation, I warmly greeted the attending physician as he came into the room. When he finished testing my blood, I asked if I was doing any better. He told me the results were the same. I inquired if this was normal. He hesitated and then told me that I had a serious infection, and it can take time for the antibiotics to work. I knew by his relatively vague response that there should be progress by now, but he didn't stay around for further questions.

It was becoming clear to me that if I didn't get better in a day or two, I'd need to start letting family and friends know what was going on. These would be very difficult phone calls, and some people would start making plans to fly west to see me; I decided to wait and see how my blood test went the following day. If there was still no improvement, I'd talk with Dr. Gale about my options.

The next day in the ICU, after a difficult, long night with little sleep, I woke up with a great deal of nervous anticipation. It was a decisive day. Breakfast helped to calm me down a bit, but it seemed like an eternity before the attending physician opened the door to my "cell" and came in to see how I was doing. He greeted me warmly and went through the process of checking the status of my blood infection. On this occasion, however, I saw a smile creep across his face. "Mr. Armstrong, we have progress to report this morning. The antibiotics are working; your infection is in decline."

My grin was much bigger than his. The infection wasn't gone, but I was on the road to recovery. The very first thing I did was call Anne and give her the good news. She screamed with joy. If all went well, we'd be back on our journey of life together. Isolation room be damned, it was the first happy day I'd spent in that lonely ICU. Those cold white walls suddenly seemed almost cheerful.

The next morning my condition improved even more, and on the seventh day in the ICU, Dr. Gale told me I no longer showed any signs of infection. He said they would need to do one more test the following day to confirm these results, but he was confident they would discharge me. He also said (to my surprise and relief) that I was now free to leave the confines of the ICU and get a little exercise walking around the hospital.

I couldn't believe it. I no longer had to stare at those clean white walls with only the TV and telephone to keep me company. I could wander about and talk to other people. As I left my room and took those first steps down the hall, I felt both humble and thankful. The doors to all the other ICU rooms were closed, but I knew that behind those doors the other patients were likely struggling with uncertainty, anxiety, and depression, just as I had.

As I exited the ICU, I had no idea where I was going. All I wanted to do was stretch my legs and get a chance to interact with someone besides my physicians and nurses. I walked down one floor and found myself in the pediatric cancer ward. Each room I passed contained a child in a bed hooked up to tubes and wires, looking visibly bored and despondent. The ward was gloomy and deathly quiet. I didn't see any visitors, nor did I see any games or other distractions to help these kids deal with being cooped up in a hospital with a deadly disease.

I immediately felt sad for these young patients. This was a time in their lives when they should be active, engaged, laughing, playing. The kids in this ward looked as if they were simply marking time, with only treatments, doctors, nurses, and disease to fill their lonely days. After battling leukemia for a month and then spending a lonely week in the ICU filled with all the uncertainty and fear associated with my bloodstream infection, I had a rough idea of what these kids were going through. I knew how important it was to have some kind of distraction to keep your mind off the disease and potential outcomes.

About halfway down the hall, I decided to stop into one of the rooms. Lying in bed, hooked up to a myriad of machines, was a boy around twelve years old. He brightened up as I entered the room. After exchanging greetings, he told me that since both his parents worked, he rarely had visitors and was very happy to have someone to talk to. He said he missed school, especially his favorite teacher. He also missed sports, which he had to stop when he was diagnosed with cancer. I told him I understood how he felt, since I was new to L.A. and was pretty much separated from all of my friends and family. We talked for almost thirty minutes, and then I wished him all the best with his care.

Down the hall I entered the room of another boy about the same age. He also told me that he didn't get many visitors and was really bored. His family consisted of only him, his mother, and a younger brother. His mother had to work and take care of his younger brother, so she couldn't visit as often as she wanted. He said it was hard facing all of this alone, and he feared his cancer treatments weren't making him any better.

I told him that I had also been scared of my cancer, especially the uncertainty both of not knowing if I was getting better or worse and of what the future would bring. However, I reassured him that there was hope. I too had been very sick, but the doctors had been able to get my cancer under control. I explained that it can take time for the treatments to work, and that he should never give up his fight to recover. He seemed encouraged by my brief personal story, or perhaps just happy to have someone to talk to and something to do besides lying in his bed alone thinking of the worst.

> " Seeing these kids stuck inside a sterile hospital room with few visitors and little to do, when they should be out enjoying their young lives, made me want to do something to help. "
>
> —MIKE ARMSTRONG

Twenty minutes into our discussion, I felt fatigue setting in. After all, I'd just spent a week in a hospital room fighting a serious bloodstream infection, and this relatively short walk proved to be a bit of a workout. So, with a handshake, a smile, and a "good luck," I left.

I slowly made my way back through the double doors and climbed the stairs that led to the ICU. I was once again facing one of those big "tomorrows," when I would learn what the rest of my life was going to look like. All signs pointed to my release, but my recent rollercoaster of disease made me cautious not to get ahead of myself. I still had one more test to confirm that I was free to leave this lonely ICU and walk back into life. Sometimes, it gets more nerve-racking the closer you get to what you desperately want, which in my case was beating the infection. I could almost smell the fresh air of freedom. However, I knew that fate could easily return me to the antiseptic isolation of the ICU.

Luckily, the following day my blood showed no infection. I'd beaten this thing and was free to leave the hospital. Now I could truly celebrate. However, the joy of knowing I'd survived was tinged with sorrow. I knew that the other patients in the ICU were not going home. They were still confined in their rooms with their disease and an uncertain future. Even more troubling were the two boys I'd met in the children's cancer ward. Unlike adults, who had at least experienced some of the fullness of life, children with cancer are just beginning their lives. This terrible disease threatened not only to take away their precious childhood but also to steal their future as teenagers, college students, husbands, and fathers.

It was clear that their endless empty days stuck in a hospital did not generate the kind of determination and hope one needs to fight cancer. These kids needed to engage in some activities to get their minds off their illness and onto something more positive. It was a difficult situation that I couldn't resolve that afternoon, but I promised myself I'd find a way to help them.

As I drove back to my condo, I thought of the many calls I wanted to make to let friends and family know I'd survived leukemia and a serious blood infection. Since only Anne, my brother, and a couple of friends even knew I was sick, my other family members and friends would likely be upset that I hadn't told them. The only way to approach this was to be completely honest. I needed to carefully explain that I had a great doctor and a solid treatment regime, and Anne and I truly believed that I was going to survive. Thus, I didn't want people to worry unnecessarily. I also had a responsibility to Hughes to keep my disease under wraps.

As expected, these were emotional calls. My daughters were especially disappointed that I hadn't told them, but in the end, they understood. Most importantly, they were all happy to know I was on the mend, and they accepted my reasons for not broadcasting my condition.

My dad, in some ways, was the easiest to talk to because he didn't make a big deal out of it. Like me, he was a "give me the facts" kind of guy. He just wanted to know that I was okay. He then shifted into talking about his golf game and his new putter. It might sound a bit insensitive, but it wasn't. It was just my dad's way. Like my mom (who had passed away a few years back), Dad was a product of a tough era, when the mentality was "if it isn't broken, don't complain, and if it is broken, fix it." In many ways I used this same approach to life, which explains my relatively pragmatic approach to my battles with cancer and my infection. These were the lessons I learned growing up, and they helped me get through a lot of difficult times.

It was truly wonderful to be able to finally share with friends and family what I'd just endured and celebrate that I had more life to live. However, I kept thinking of the children in the pediatric cancer ward at the UCLA cancer center and their difficult, lonely battle. I knew I had to do something to help them. So, I decided to call a friend, Danny Bakewell, who worked in real estate in the L.A. area. His daughter Sabriya had battled leukemia and lost. Thus, Danny knew firsthand how difficult it was for a child to fight cancer. Perhaps he had some ideas of how I could help.

I got Danny on the phone and told him about my leukemia experiences. He was sad to hear I had been ill but delighted I'd been discharged and was healthy again. I once again expressed my sympathies on his losing Sabriya, as I knew how much he missed her. Then I told him about my walk down the hall of the children's cancer ward and how sad it was to see these kids fighting cancer with nothing to occupy their time but doctors and disease.

Danny told me he knew the situation all too well. He had

spent a lot of time in hospitals visiting Sabriya during her leu-kemia battle and had been greatly disturbed by the loneliness and boredom associated with cancer and cancer wards. In fact, the experience had such an effect on him that he had done something about it—he had designed a kid's play station that fit on a standard hospital cart, so nurses could wheel it right up to the bedside. He called it Sabriya's Castle, and it included a TV, movies, games, and story tapes. It didn't replace family or other visitors, but at least it took some of the focus away from cancer, boredom, and loneliness for the kids in his daughter's cancer ward.

I almost yelled, "Danny, that is a terrific idea!"

We immediately agreed to jointly produce a number of Sa-briya's Castles. We set up an assembly and testing space, hired staff, and started calling hospitals. Every hospital we contacted told us they wanted units as soon as we could deliver. We agreed to cover the cost of around $500 to build each system, and the hospitals agreed to cover the ongoing maintenance.

> " Cancer can make you reflect to the point that it
> makes you depressed; or, it can change the way
> you hope for things. This opportunity to reflect
> can be a gift, if you use it correctly. "
>
> —DR. WILLIAM NELSON

During the seven years I worked at Hughes, we provided Sabriya's Castles to children's cancer wards in hospitals through-out L.A. Each ward (roughly twenty kids) got multiple castles. I visited several of these hospitals and witnessed firsthand how these relatively simple entertainment centers boosted kids' spirits, making the otherwise boring and lonely cancer unit a little more fun. The positive reactions we got from the children, nurses, doctors, and staff brought Danny and me enormous satisfaction.

In 2012, Gillian Lichota found a lump in her right breast when she was undergoing hormonal IVF treatments in order to have her first child. She was in her early thirties and nine weeks pregnant when her doctor told her that she had stage 3 breast cancer that had spread into her lymph nodes.

She underwent an extensive eight-hour surgery to have both her lymph nodes and her breast removed and breast reconstruction. Since she was still pregnant, she had to make the agonizing decision either to start chemotherapy right away or wait until after she had given birth. Her doctor assured her that the pregnancy had progressed far enough that her unborn child would not be affected by the chemotherapy, but it was still a lot to manage both physically and emotionally.

"When you are first diagnosed with cancer, there are all these things you have to do. You're inundated. You really feel like you're in this dark valley and there's this large mountain in front of you that you have to climb, which is the cancer mountain, with all the treatments and surgeries and doctor appointments, and it interferes with your life, your career, and all the things that you love to do."

Instead of letting depression and despair get the better of her, she managed to find the hope she needed to get on with her treatments. She also set a goal for herself. She decided that after she climbed her analogous mountain of treatments, she'd climb a real mountain, specifically, Mount Kilimanjaro, in Tanzania—something that had long been on her bucket list.

Gillian went through the chemotherapy and hormone therapy and had a healthy baby boy. One month after her son was born, she went through a different form of aggressive chemotherapy, radiation, and more surgeries, and then she was finally finished with her treatments.

All of this, understandably, took a toll on Gillian's physical and emotional health. She'd always been active and was both an outdoor enthusiast and a triathlete. However, because of all the treatments and downtime, she'd gained thirty pounds, experienced extreme fatigue, and her muscles had atrophied. In addition, having her lymph nodes removed greatly restricted her range of motion. Furthermore, hormonal therapy had given her severe joint pain and stiffness and nerve damage in her feet and hands that felt like constant, painful pins and needles. She was clearly in no condition to hike to an elevation of 19,341 feet above sea level.

Unwilling to give up and give in, she found a group of health and wellness experts (yoga instructors, fitness trainers, nutritionists, as well as acupuncture and massage therapists), who helped her address what her treatments had done to her general health. This not only enabled her to get her body back in shape so she could climb Mount Kilimanjaro, but she believes it also helped her achieve long-term remission.

"The climb to the summit of Mount Kilimanjaro was awesome. I went with one of my close friends, just the two of us. On the final day of our ascent, we left base camp on a full moon at 10:30 at night. It was not easy. You're going up, up, up. You're climbing and losing oxygen as you gain altitude, and the air gets really thin. You're conserving your oxygen, so you cannot talk, which gives you a lot of time to yourself. It was very cathartic, because you're in your own head and thinking about a lot of things in your life. I was thinking about all I have been through, what mattered to me most in life, and where I wanted to go with my life. We arrived at the summit at 6 in the morning. Everything was illuminated. Everything seemed so clear to me. It was brilliant."

Gillian says her two dogs had both died shortly before that climb, and she decided to bring their ashes to the top of Mount Kilimanjaro since they had always gone hiking with her. As she scattered her dogs' ashes on the summit with the sun rising over Africa, she became overwhelmed with emotion. "I just kept sobbing and crying. It was minus five degrees up there, very cold. Two guys came by and said 'Are you OK?' I had snot and tears running down my face. I said, 'I am okay, just so proud to be here.'"

When she came back from Africa, she shared her story with her oncologist, who thought Gillian might be able to help other patients find hope and purpose in their journey with breast cancer. Gillian agreed to meet with a few of the oncologist's young female patients and was amazed at how these women shared many of the age-specific challenges, fears, and concerns that she had with her cancer. This gave birth to the idea of creating a support program that could help young women deal with the challenges associated with having breast cancer. She was not exactly sure what that program would be, but a seed had been planted.

Five years after her first experience with cancer and her inspiring ascent to the summit of Mount Kilimanjaro, breast cancer returned to Gillian's life, only this time she was stage 4, which is essentially incurable.

"For the first time in my life, I entered a really deep, deep, dark place for three weeks. I could not make a decision, I could not get out of bed, I just thought, 'Oh my God. I'm going to die this time. This is it for me. This is it.'"

One of her triathlon girlfriends called Gillian and tried to get her out of her slump by inviting her to come to the pool and train. "I sat there on the end of my bed and literally cursed her in my mind, thinking, 'Are you crazy?' I told her 'Thank you, but no thank you,' and ended the call. I sat there on the end of my bed thinking about all that had happened. . . . And then I said to myself, 'You know what? I'm going to that pool.'"

Gillian showed up at the pool and had one of her best swims in a very long time. "I got into that pool and thought, 'Yes. This is it. This is my life. Cancer's not going to define me. It's not going to win.'"

At that point, Gillian decided to move forward with her idea of helping other young women to feel empowered and find purpose, strength, and hope in their battle with breast cancer and formed the nonprofit organization iRise Above Foundation. Over the years since then, Gillian's cancer has remained under control, and her organization has flourished.

The iRise Above Foundation connects participants with a number of health experts who help these women address areas in their lives—diet, exercise, emotional state, spiritual state—that are negatively affecting their health and happiness. The program also hosts a number of wellness retreats where participants enjoy a variety of healthful activities and commune with nature.

Gillian says doctors don't pay enough attention to the emotional aspects of cancer, like the need for self-empowerment, hope, and purpose. Cancer patients desperately need hope. The label "cancer" can bring doom and gloom, but cancer also provides an opportunity for you to create positive change in your life.

She says a sense of purpose keeps you positive. It helps you feel you still have a lot to give back to the world. "The moment you start feeling you have nothing to contribute, it's a nail in your coffin. You have to keep thinking 'I am still worthy. I still have a voice, a purpose. I get to choose the life I want to live. I can change lives and make a difference.'"

Gillian has zero plans for leaving this Earth anytime soon. However, because she knows that having metastatic cancer means her health could deteriorate at any moment, she prefers to take advantage of the time she has to "live fully, love deeply, and have a positive impact on others."

"Every day is a gift. I don't know what the future brings. But I'm okay today."

Chapter 11

IN 1998, ANNE AND I said goodbye to California and moved to New Jersey, where I took a position as CEO of AT&T before eventually retiring and moving back to a house we owned in Darien, Connecticut. We'd built the house in 1973, when I worked at IBM's White Plains office. Of all the houses we'd lived in as my career moved us around the country and the world, we'd kept our place in Darien because it always felt like home.

Now that I was back on the East Coast, I decided to reconnect with Johns Hopkins University in Baltimore, Maryland. I'd first started working with the university in 1981. IBM's then-CEO, Frank Carey, had asked the company's executives to seek out and establish relationships with the nation's best academic research institutions in order to stay on the cutting edge of technology. Many leading research universities—MIT, Harvard, the University of Michigan, the University of California, Berkeley—were already engaged with IBM, but Johns Hopkins was not.

Jack Kuehler, one of IBM's executives and my good friend, knew some of the folks at Johns Hopkins. I contacted him, and we visited the university together. After a series of meetings and discussions, I established both an IBM partnership and a personal relationship with the university.

Back then, my IBM interests centered primarily on the Johns Hopkins Applied Physics Laboratory and the Whiting School of Engineering. However, given how thankful I was to have survived leukemia and my blood infection, I started looking at ways to support Johns Hopkins' medical school and hospitals. As my involvement with Hopkins increased, I became a member of the Board of Trustees at Johns Hopkins University and later the chairman of Johns Hopkins Medicine Health System Corporation and Hospital.

Around this time, I was both saddened and inspired by another victim of cancer whose life and purpose had been profoundly changed by the disease. Fred Scholtz was a good friend who lived near us in Darien. He and I were avid tennis players, who regularly played each other throughout the summer.

One evening, Fred called to tell me that he'd been diagnosed with pancreatic cancer. I couldn't believe what I was hearing. Just the other day we were playing tennis, and he seemed fine. In fact, Fred was one of the healthiest, most active people I knew. He used to joke that he hadn't had a physical exam since he weighed eight pounds, four ounces. Pancreatic cancer is one of the more difficult cancers, in that only 9 percent of patients are expected to live more than five years after first diagnosis (see Sources Cited, ACS, Survival Rates for Pancreatic Cancer 2015).

Knowing that I was active at Johns Hopkins Medicine, Fred asked if I could recommend doctors who might help him better understand and treat his disease. I immediately connected him with some of the institution's leading oncologists. For eight days Fred met with Hopkins' brightest and best. Unfortunately, his cancer was untreatable, and they told him he likely had only about nine months to live.

Fred had a lot of life still in him and wasn't ready to throw in the towel. An amateur photographer who had won numerous awards over the years, he had always wanted to travel the world with his camera and create a special album that he could share with family and friends. So, with cancer and with camera in hand, Fred set off on his "life journey," which lasted six months. He went to extraordinary lengths to capture beautiful photos of wildlife, landscapes, and people from around the world. This trip truly celebrated Fred's passion for life—a life he knew he would soon be leaving.

Fred's doctors had given him an array of medications to help him cope with his advancing disease. However, the best elixir for Fred's condition was his tenacity and courage, and the excitement and wonder he had for his great adventure, all of which seemed to keep his disease at bay.

> " I believe that when you compare those with cancer and those who have no evidence of any type of disease, the group that has cancer often has a higher quality of life. "
>
> **—DR. WILLIAM NELSON**

When he returned home, he feverishly sorted through his photographs and created the associated text for the book. He called it "Favorite Places" and made arrangements to have it published. It took him several months to complete the book, during which his condition steadily worsened, leaving him no choice but to finally enter a hospice care facility.

Once in hospice, his cancer went into high gear. As a result, Fred's doctors told him he likely had only a few more days to live and should start arranging his affairs. I visited Fred every day and marveled at both his resilience and his acceptance that his time had come. In spite of his impending death and the agony associated with pancreatic cancer, Fred kept his head high and never lost sight of his final desire—getting his book completed. Unfortunately, it had not yet arrived from the publisher, as planned.

Fred was never one to ask favors. However, during one of my visits, he told me how important it was for him to hold the book in his hands and see it before he left this world. He asked if I could somehow ask the publisher to speed completion and delivery. I told him I would do whatever I could do to make that happen.

After many calls, I managed to find someone at the publishing company who could help with my request. He told me the book was finished; they just hadn't gotten around to sending it out. When I explained Fred's condition and the importance of getting the book to him as soon as possible, he said they'd arrange to have a copy of the book picked that afternoon so that it could be delivered the following morning.

I was in front of the hospice facility at 7:30 a.m., cup of coffee in hand, waiting. At 7:45 the FedEx truck pulled up, and the driver jumped out with the shipment in hand. I thanked him profusely and opened the package while walking to Fred's room. I went directly to his bedside and handed Fred his book. With a huge smile he began turning pages and sharing with me some of the priceless travel moments he'd experienced on this wonderful journey.

Sadly, Fred died several days later. However, I will always remember how he chose to make the most of the last days pursuing a lifelong dream. A copy of his book sits proudly in the living room of our home in Darien and is a beautiful reminder of how he celebrated life even as he faced a deadly disease.

Cancer dramatically changes our perspective on life and what we want to do with it. Many cancer patients, including myself, have experienced this change. In many ways, it's the silver lining that comes with that dark cloud of cancer. When we fear that our days might be numbered, time becomes much more precious and there's a strong desire to use it wisely, with meaning and purpose.

PATIENT STORY: *Leslie Ries*

Leslie Ries was diagnosed with breast cancer in 2004, when she was forty-eight. "I was diagnosed with a fast-growing triple negative breast cancer and tested positive for the genetic mutation known as BRCA1." These two "risk" factors greatly increased her chances of having continuing problems with breast cancer and also for getting ovarian cancer. "Many patients with triple negative breast cancer don't make it past the first five years."

Leslie had a lumpectomy, chemotherapy, and radiation therapy. Given her high risk factors, she also decided on a double mastectomy, but instead of getting artificial implants, she elected to have tissue and blood vessels transferred from her backside to her chest to serve as implants. This was a much more extensive surgical procedure, but she says it was safer than artificial implants, which can have long-term risks. She also had her ovaries removed because of the high risk for ovarian cancer associated with BRCA1. In total, she had four months of chemotherapy and nine surgical procedures over an eighteen-month period. "All of those treatments gave me a lot of time to think about many things."

Leslie was a partner in a law firm when she was diagnosed. During her treatment, she worked when she could. When she was too sick to work, she spent time at home with her two daughters—one was in her last year of high school, and the other worked nearby and visited often.

"If I didn't have cancer, I wouldn't have been home as much for my daughter in her senior year. We tried to look at the positive side of what we were getting out of this experience. It was horrific, but we were trying to think of the positive."

After fighting the disease for a while, she decided to leave the firm and start her own practice so that she would have more time to focus on other things that were important to her. "I loved my job, but I'd been doing this a long time. It was time to do things differently and do different things."

From the very early stage of her treatment, Leslie had an intense desire to help other patients. One of the things she did was make thank-you cards for cancer patients to give to people who had helped them during their treatment.

She also tried to help women manage the trauma of losing their hair by encouraging them to donate their hair to make wigs (before it falls out). "Interestingly, many women worry more about losing their hair than their breasts." She says that by donating their hair, when and how to lose it becomes their decision. "They own it instead of it owning them."

Leslie's cancer was likely hereditary: her grandmother died of metastatic breast cancer at a young age. This family history of cancer made her especially concerned for her two daughters. She wanted to do something to protect them from also getting cancer, so she talked to her oncologist. "I kept saying, 'What can I do? Tell me what I can do to help.'"

Her oncologist told her about the importance of prevention research and how researchers are always struggling to get funding. Leslie decided that helping raise money for prevention research would be a great way for her to focus her energies and also help future generations. Over the years since she started that work, she has helped researchers raise millions of dollars to fund their work.

Leslie says that researchers are looking at a number of ways to predict and prevent cancer, such as looking at whether the specific cell structure of women's breasts might make them more susceptible to cancer, or developing a blood test that identifies people with breast cancer at an early stage, when it's still treatable.

Both Leslie's daughters have the BRCA1 mutation, so they get MRIs twice a year, and they regularly get breast exams. Her older daughter now has a five-year-old son. When she was 32, she decided that she didn't want to risk getting cancer and not be around for him. She had a prophylactic double mastectomy and reconstructive surgery and also had her ovaries removed. "You know what? I have one wonderful son and I'm here. Guess what? He's perfect . . . I don't want to worry that I'll get breast cancer by waiting to take this action."

Leslie is very excited about the future of cancer prevention. She sees a time where we can look at entire families and predict who is at risk and how to approach and minimize that risk. She sees this not just for breast cancer but for all cancers.

Chapter 12

I WAS LUCKY to have had a treatable form of leukemia. However, I was not free and clear. I knew my leukemia could return at any moment and it was always in the back of my mind. Therefore, I made sure to visit my doctors regularly and have my blood routinely tested. It was with a good deal of apprehension that I showed up for these blood tests, and huge relief bordering on outright excitement when I heard the words, "Your blood counts are stable."

My health checkups didn't stop there. I also had regular prostate-specific antigen (PSA) tests to check for prostate cancer. This disease is predominately associated with older men—as I was in my early 60s, I was in the prime target zone. However, I also knew it could be successfully treated if detected early (see Sources Cited, ACS, About Prostate Cancer 2019).

My prostate physician was Dr. Patrick Walsh, whom I'd met at Johns Hopkins when I was scaling up my involvement with the institution. I was very fortunate to have connected with him, as he is one of the world's top prostate cancer specialists and urology surgeons.

All went well in my life and health until 2003, when my PSA count went from negligible to 4. This was a big jump and cause for concern. Dr. Walsh ordered a biopsy, which extracted tiny tissue samples of my prostate for the lab to examine for cancer. To my relief, the results were negative. Dr. Walsh explained that high PSA does not always indicate prostate cancer, but could be due to other causes that are not life threatening. He said the only way to confirm was to take a tissue sample; if my PSA numbers continued to rise, we'd do a second biopsy.

A year later, my PSA count had increased from 4 to 8. Having my numbers double in twelve months to this level was an even stronger indication of potential prostate cancer than the previous jump from 0 to 4. Dr. Walsh ordered another biopsy, and to our relief and surprise, the results were negative. He once again explained that this kind of rise in PSA count could also occur in patients who do not have prostate cancer, although the percentage of men in this category is very small.

The following year, 2005, my PSA count went from 8 to 17. In spite of the lack of evidence from my biopsies, both Dr. Walsh and I suspected that these high numbers likely indicated that something was going on with my prostate. He ordered a much more aggressive biopsy, which meant increasing the number of tissue samples significantly. This time, he found cancer. Luckily, it appeared to be relatively minor, affecting only 5 percent of one of these tissue samples.

In spite of this being "low profile," Dr. Walsh recommended a radical prostatectomy. This procedure removes the entire prostate and any other associated infected tissue to prevent the cancer from spreading to the rest of my body.

It was a troubling discovery to learn that cancer was back in my life. However, since the snips indicated that it was not extensive, we likely detected it early and thus it was treatable. That being said, given the tough battle I had fought with leukemia and the resulting blood infection, I was more than a little concerned. One cancer in a lifetime is enough for any person. When I returned home to Connecticut that evening after seeing Dr. Walsh, I shared the prostate cancer diagnosis with Anne.

She was both alarmed and concerned that cancer was back in my life and that it might have been there for three years, while my PSA number had been going up. The bigger question that troubled us was: If it had been growing throughout those years, would it still be treatable? We talked for hours about all of the possible scenarios regarding my diagnosis; we even wondered if it might be related to my leukemia.

I knew that the only way to manage all this uncertainty was to remain hopeful and look at the facts: (1) my PSA counts were alarmingly high, (2) my biopsy suggested I had some level of prostate cancer, (3) Dr. Walsh was one of the best urology surgeons in the world and an expert on prostate cancer, and (4) I wouldn't know anything more until Dr. Walsh opened me up and took a look.

So, I scheduled the surgery and went into the operating room hoping for the best. Instead of letting my mind race with frustration and anger at having to deal with another major health issue, I reminded myself that life is full of challenges. I'd faced a lot of them already, and I'd likely face many more. The important thing was not to dwell on the negative but try to make the best out of a tough situation.

Looking back over my life and career, one of the biggest challenges I encountered was at Hughes Electronics when I thought I might have to lay off almost a quarter of our workforce of more than 80,000 employees. In the early nineties, after the Soviet Union had collapsed and the Cold War ended, the need for our satellites and other defense technology diminished considerably, and the US government significantly reduced the extent of the contracts it had with Hughes.

I faced a difficult decision. We could downsize and merge with some of the other struggling defense contractors, or find a way to adapt, grow, and survive. After considerable thought, I chose to find a positive way out of our dilemma that would not only preserve jobs but also help Hughes see this crisis as an opportunity, not a failure.

I met with our leadership team, and we all agreed that we needed to adjust the company's focus and significantly expand into non-defense-related commercial products and markets. Our initial attention turned to a relatively small research and development project at Hughes that was looking into using our satellite technology to broadcast high-bandwidth digital video.

In the early 1990s, television in America was delivered as an analog signal via antenna or cable. By using large-bandwidth digital technology delivered via satellite, we could theoretically revolutionize television. We'd not only provide more channels and higher definition images but also eliminate the need for both antennas and cables. Most importantly, we were confident we could deliver this exciting new product at approximately the same price as cable television. Several industry experts and companies outside of Hughes were exploring similar technology, but no one had announced anything. If we successfully launched a digital satellite television service ahead of the competition, we could get an edge on the market that could begin to offset the decline of our defense business.

After many meetings and debates, we decided to take the gamble and move ahead with the idea. This was one of the most critical decisions of my career, but I was confident it was the best option and worth the risk. We assembled a team to aggressively develop the technology with the goal of making Hughes the "national cable company in the sky." We called it DirecTV and put a business plan together to persuade the board of directors at both Hughes and our parent company, General Motors.

There was no question we faced some big challenges: (1) DirecTV would cost roughly one billion dollars in upfront investment; (2) we had to develop local retailing and service locations and train people to sell both the dish on the roof and the television programming in the living room; (3) we needed to develop the financial and logistical systems to effectively support a national commercial business; and (4) we would need sales, marketing, and advertising strategies for both local and national markets.

On the positive side, we projected that we would have ten million DirecTV subscribers over the next ten years, which would translate into a very good return on investment. Both the Hughes and GM boards approved our plan. In the end, we not only recovered our investment and made considerable profits to offset our losses, we also revolutionized the way the world watches and thinks about television. Today, DirecTV (which AT&T later purchased and rebranded as DIRECTV) has more than thirty million subscribers.

> " Hope is essential. Everybody's really focused on medicine, and hope doesn't get a lot of attention. "
> —CHRISTINE HOGDON, A PERSON WITH CANCER

Life is full of adversity, and it comes in many forms. No matter what happens, no matter how bad things appear, it's essential to maintain the hope and conviction that you can achieve a positive outcome. Challenge can bring out the best in us; we often don't even know what we're made of until we're put to the test. I've seen this time and time again in my life and career, and also with regard to the many challenges I faced with cancer. My journey through cancer was not only about beating the disease but also about maintaining hope and not letting cancer define me or own me.

One very personal story that speaks to this involves my father, who got leukemia when he was ninety-one, many years after I battled the disease.

Music was one of my dad's biggest passions. For years, he had played drums in a small jazz band, which performed on weekends. When his days became numbered, and we were packing a few of the belongings he wanted to take to hospice, he asked me to include his snare drum, cymbals, drum sticks, and brushes. I couldn't help wondering why, but I didn't ask; I just packed them.

During my dad's first four days in hospice, he was occupied with the myriad of treatments necessary to relieve his pain and discomfort. However, on the fifth day, Don, a good friend and the saxophone player in Dad's former band called to say he was coming to visit. My dad told him to bring his saxophone.

> "Hope is a calibration. Figure out what you're hoping for. That might change over time, but figure out what you're hoping for."
>
> —DR. WILLIAM NELSON

That afternoon, to everyone's surprise and delight, Dad and Don set up the drums and cymbals in the hallway. They played a few standard tunes and then took requests from doctors, nurses, and patients for over an hour. Afterward, my father returned to his room, went right to sleep, and never woke up.

PATIENT STORY: Christine Hogdon

Christine Hogdon's battle with metastatic breast cancer has taken her down a long and arduous path of difficult treatments, associated disease, and troubling uncertainty. For many, this would be too much to bear. However, instead of letting it destroy her life, Christine found hope and purpose and decided to transform these challenges into something positive.

Her many years working in the science field as a conservation biologist gave her a unique ability to understand the complex ever-changing world of research and clinical trials. So, she decided to become a patient advocate and use her skills to help other cancer patients locate and enroll in the clinical trials best suited to their disease, personal needs, and goals.

Christine started small, but became more and more active as she began attending advocacy conferences. She started taking time off of work, first just one month and then more, until the whole thing snowballed. Now she says it seems as if she's always working, but she doesn't mind. "I love it! I'm kind of known in the community as the clinical trial guru for metastatic breast cancer. I'm helping the most vulnerable patients, and I can't imagine anything more rewarding."

Christine still does this mostly on her own, with very little financial help. She says patients often offer to donate, but she feels uncomfortable taking money from them. The only support she receives comes from grants that cover her travel expenses to conferences.

Patients find Christine via doctor recommendations, the internet, and social media. "I get e-mails and messages from people I've never met in my life. People find out that I know about trials, and they come straight to me asking for help." She works with people from all over the United States and has even had patients from England and Scotland.

Christine says she often works with people who are near the end of their lives and are coming to her with few remaining options. "It is particularly difficult to find a trial for which these patients will qualify, but I have to constantly remind myself, it's the doctor's job to save patients, it's my job to give them hope."

Chapter 13

As a fall sun glimmered through the window of my room at Johns Hopkins Hospital the morning following my prostate cancer surgery, one thing struck me as a bit odd. Dr. Walsh had not stopped by my room the previous evening after the surgery. By that time, I'd known Dr. Walsh for a number of years and was pretty sure that he almost always visits his patients post-surgery. I could only assume that he had to attend to other more critical patients or perform an emergency procedure.

Shortly after I finished my breakfast, Dr. Walsh finally came in to see me. As soon as he entered the room, I knew something was wrong. Unlike our other meetings, which were usually jovial, on this morning he was noticeably frowning and rather serious in his bedside manner. After a compulsory "Good morning Mike, are you feeling okay?," he looked me in the eye and said "We had a different outcome than expected."

He told me that when he opened me up, he found that the cancer had grown out of the prostate and into the surrounding pelvic area. Instead of a routine one-hour prostate removal surgery, I'd been in the operating room for more than four hours. He'd removed the prostate and a good-sized tumor, but surgery alone could not remove all the cancer cells. The good news was it was contained in my pelvic area and had not metastasized. However, it was significantly advanced.

To say I was shocked would be a huge understatement. I'd expected to hear that the surgery was successful, my cancer gone, and I'd be going home the next day. What I learned was that they could not remove all my cancer; it might spread to other parts of my body, and it was potentially life threatening. My head was full of questions once again. How did this happen? What were my odds for survival? Was this a death sentence? But all I could muster was, "What do we do now?"

Dr. Walsh began outlining the treatment strategy. He said I would need external beam radiation therapy, five days a week for nine weeks, and intense hormonal therapy for two to three years.

External beam radiation therapy aims high-energy particle waves directly at cancer cells. This damages the cancer's DNA, which prevents these cells from dividing—the idea being that if the cancer cannot reproduce, it will eventually die off. A downside of radiation therapy is that it also kills normal cells, which can result in various side effects, depending on what part of the body is targeted. Doctors are very careful to make sure that collateral cell damage is limited to what the body can handle. In my case, Dr. Walsh assured me that the only noticeable side effect I'd have from the radiation would be some soreness and fatigue.

Hormonal therapy starves the cancer by reducing or eliminating the production (and thus the availability) of hormones called androgens (such as testosterone), which prostate cancer needs to survive. The big downside of hormonal therapy is that the human body needs androgens to maintain general health. Low androgen levels can cause serious negative side effects, including insulin resistance, mood swings, fatigue, memory loss, impotence, liver damage, bone fractures, and loss of muscle mass and strength.

As unpleasant and long as this list sounds, any one or combination of these "side effects" was preferable to death, which was likely if the prostate cancer metastasized.

Dr. Walsh explained that I could start hormonal therapy soon, but I'd have to wait ninety days before starting radiation treatment to allow time for my prostate to heal after surgery. In order to monitor whether the cancer was growing, I'd need to have a PSA test every thirty days. He concluded by referring me to one of Hopkins' best radiation oncologists, Dr. Theodore DeWeese. He also apologized for not visiting me post-surgery, saying that he was upset that he had misjudged the extent of the cancer and needed time to carefully consider my options before meeting with me. I replied that I also needed time to absorb what was happening to me, but I appreciated his empathy and honesty.

> " Cancer can be a lot of doom and gloom, and patients desperately need to find hope. "
>
> —GILLIAN LICHOTA, A PERSON WITH CANCER

After Dr. Walsh left my room, I started processing the disturbing reality that I was once again in a serious battle with an advanced cancer that could take my life. Equally disturbing was the realization that I was also again the victim of a wrong diagnosis. If Dr. Walsh had been able to detect my cancer when my PSA count first started increasing, he would likely have removed the prostate before the cancer progressed. As it was, the cancer had grown outside of my prostate and could continue to spread to other parts of my body and potentially kill me.

I understood this was not Dr. Walsh's fault. He was using the best tools he had available and following the guidelines explicitly. The problem was that my cancer was focused on the front of my prostate, which is shielded by my pelvic bone and hard to access in a biopsy. In these cases, PSA numbers can be high while biopsies show no evidence of disease.

For now, however, I had to forget about the past and focus on hope and a plan. My first order of business was to review the facts: (1) I had prostate cancer in my pelvic area that could

spread to other parts of my body; (2) it was difficult for doctors
to know exactly where it might spread and to what extent other
parts of my body might be affected; (3) my only options were
radiation and hormonal treatments, with no guarantee of success and survival; and (4) I could not start radiation therapy for
ninety days.

I was back in a world of medical uncertainty that was even
vaguer and more disturbing than what I'd experienced with leukemia. Was my cancer curable now? Would it still be curable in
ninety days, when I was scheduled to start radiation treatment?
How would I respond to the radiation and hormonal therapy?
Was I fighting for only a few more years of life, with little hope
of longer-term survival? Was there some new clinical trial or
treatment available (as I had with leukemia) that might provide
hope for sustained life?

Unfortunately, only thirty days after my surgery, my PSA
levels tripled. Whatever cancer Dr. Walsh had been unable to
remove was now aggressively growing and spreading. In spite
of this, I still had to wait sixty days before I could start my radiation treatments. It was a crushing blow, but one I just had to
deal with.

PATIENT STORY: *David Gobin*

In April of 2008, shortly after being diagnosed with lung cancer,
David Gobin had part of his lung surgically removed and then
enrolled in a clinical trial that combined chemotherapy with
radiation. Unfortunately, the trial did not work, and they found
spots on his kidney and liver, as well as a tumor attached to the
pleural membrane that lines the inside of his chest wall. He had
another operation and more chemotherapy and radiation, but
again, the tumors returned.

"My oncologist at the time simply said, 'Sorry.' I could see she had been crying."

At the time, David was trying any clinical trial that came up, but he was running out of options. "I was willing to do anything they suggested. I was on one trial where I had to go to Hopkins six days a week for a shot in the stomach. My stomach was so bruised, they were running out of places to inject me."

In October of 2010, his oncologist told him there weren't any more treatments she could recommend and offered to give him something just to keep him comfortable. David says that was the first time he thought really seriously about the possibility that cancer might kill him. "It was especially hard on my wife. She cried a lot. I'd say to myself, 'What is she crying for? I'm the one who's dying!' Then I realized, wait a minute, I'm going to be gone, and she'll still be stuck here. I get the easy out."

Just when David thought his luck had finally run out, his oncologist found an immunotherapy trial that she thought might work for him. "They weren't really expecting a whole lot of results. The trial was mostly focused on dosage and side effects, but despite that, I said, 'Just put me in. If it works, it works.'" David figured he was pretty much a lab rat. This drug was probably not going to cure him, and it could possibly even kill him. "I didn't care. I was kind of thrilled. What did I have to lose?"

The first CAT scan David had after starting the trial showed that his tumors were growing, but in spite of that, he stayed on the trial.

"After the second CAT scan, I got a call from my oncologist, who said, 'It's shrinking.' My reply was simply, 'Oh?' To which she answered, 'Well, aren't you excited?' I remember saying, 'Well, I don't know what that means. I still have cancer, right?,' and she told me again, 'But it's shrinking. It's never shrunk before. This stuff looks like it might work on you.'"

The trial lasted for two years. During that time, David's tumors kept shrinking, and the spots on his kidney and liver also disappeared. Then he had to stop.

"That was what I'd signed up for. I couldn't stay on the drug. They wanted to see what happens after you get off it. I told my oncologist, 'The only reason I'm alive is that you are giving me this stuff. Why can't I have more?' But I signed up for the study, and those were the rules. So I had to live with it." The last time he took the drug was near the end of 2010. Since then he hasn't taken anything for his cancer, and his tumors have stayed the same size. By the time this book was written (more than a decade after his first diagnosis), his cancer was considered chronic.

David says that being a police officer made him pretty resilient. "I just kept on going, like the Energizer Bunny. They'd tell me I've got three months to live, three months passed by and I'd say, 'Now what?' Then they'd say, 'Well, you have another three months.' And then it was one year and I'd say, 'Okay, I'll just live year to year.' That was in 2008, eleven years ago."

David is grateful for the many years and experiences he has had since he was first diagnosed, especially attending his son's wedding. "I was so happy I got to see that. I lived for that." He says that his cancer journey, while difficult, opened up his life in positive ways that he'd never experienced. Before his cancer he wasn't a very sociable person. "When you work as a cop on the street you've got to be tough. You can't say please and thank you—it doesn't work. I had quite a few fights just because people looked at me too long."

Cancer changed all that, and he ended up getting involved in a lot of cancer-related activities. He was on a number of televised programs, including an appearance on a celebrity cancer TV fundraiser called *Stand Up To Cancer*. He also raised money for the lung cancer support group LUNGevity. In addition, he took time out to speak with newly diagnosed patients to help give them hope so they could better deal with what they were going through. "Lung cancer patients think it's a death sentence.

Honest to God, it took me many years and tears to realize that maybe it's not a death sentence."

David says that cancer even brought him and his wife closer, and they spend almost all their time together now. "I can't take any chances and waste time, because tomorrow I might not be here." He tries to look more on the positive side of his cancer experience than the negative. "I don't dwell on what cancer did *to* me. It's what cancer has done *for* me. And it has done a lot for me."

Cancer even turned him into a "hugger." "Back when I was a cop, I didn't like it when anyone put their hands on me. You touch me, you go to jail. Now I've learned that I like to hug. 'Hugs and drugs against cancer.' That should be my motto!"

Chapter 14

WHEN I ARRIVED BACK HOME in Connecticut, Anne and I agreed that it would be a good idea to take a break from everything and relax, reflect, and store up some energy for my upcoming radiation treatments. So, we packed our bags and headed out to our house in Telluride, Colorado, which we'd built in the early 1990s.

Our flight touched down in Telluride around noon. As Anne and I drove the twenty minutes up the winding road to our mountain home, the fresh air and 9,000-foot altitude gave me a much-needed mental and emotional break from all the stress I'd been experiencing from my second "round" with cancer.

As I carried our luggage from the car to the house, I experienced a little shortness of breath, which I chalked up to elevation change. I'd just traveled from sea level, and it usually took me a day or two to acclimate to the lower oxygen levels at high altitude. That night however, my shortness of breath intensified and I repeatedly woke up struggling to breathe. Eventually, I got out of bed and searched for a portable canister of oxygen I kept in the house for altitude sickness. I had never needed it before, but on this night, I couldn't get to sleep without it.

The next morning, my breathing got even worse, and I spent most of the day with the oxygen canister close at hand. By lunchtime, I started to wonder if perhaps my shortness of breath was due to something more serious than just the change in altitude. After lunch, feeling exhausted, I retreated to my favorite easy chair in my office and tried to relax. However, my breathing issues only got worse, until I was literally gasping for air. As I started to lose consciousness, I managed to squeak out a desperate cry for help.

Anne ran into the office and saw me collapsed in the chair, unresponsive. She immediately called 911. Talking and poking, she managed to arouse me and continued to feed me oxygen. In twenty minutes, the ambulance arrived at the house. The medics came upstairs, slapped a proper oxygen mask on my face, laid me on the stretcher, and drove me down the mountain to the Telluride Medical Center—a small emergency medical care facility in town.

By the time we arrived at the clinic my breathing had gotten a little better, but I still needed the oxygen mask. The doctor who examined me was a specialist in altitude sickness. I explained to him that I had recently undergone surgery for prostate cancer and was on hormonal therapy. In spite of this, he concluded that my breathing problem was due to altitude sickness. I respected his expertise, but I was not convinced. I'd been happily hiking, biking, skiing, and playing golf in Telluride for more than sixteen years and had never experienced anything close to this.

I passed the remaining afternoon hours resting in the clinic. My condition slowly improved, and I no longer felt as if I was going to pass out. However, I still periodically needed oxygen to help me breathe. As it was getting late in the afternoon and the medical center would soon be closing, I had to make a decision. Plan A: Drive sixty-five miles to the nearest hospital in Montrose, Colorado, for an overnight stay and more tests, or Plan B: Head back to my Telluride home and hope my condition improved.

In spite of the doctor's diagnosis, I was pretty sure there was something else affecting my lungs besides altitude sickness, something that was most likely related to my cancer or treatments. So I chose Plan C: Head to Johns Hopkins in Baltimore as soon as possible and meet with Dr. DeWeese. He knew my medical history and was better equipped to find out what was happening to me. If he couldn't figure it out, I was sure someone else at Johns Hopkins would. I picked up some extra portable oxygen canisters at the clinic and then began making arrangements to go to Baltimore the following day.

I went to bed that night in Telluride thinking about my breathing difficulties, advanced prostate cancer, impending radiation treatments, and all the side effects associated with hormonal therapy. How would I survive and cope with all of this combined? And what were the possible outcomes? Would all of this be too much for my sixty-five-year-old body and mind? As I drifted in and out of a stressful night's sleep, a scary thought reared its ugly head. Had my cancer spread to my lungs? None of the doctors at Johns Hopkins or the Telluride clinic had talked about potential lung cancer.

Anne and I took off from Telluride at half past seven in the morning, oxygen canisters in hand. When I eventually arrived at Johns Hopkins, I was admitted to an ICU room that would be my home until the doctors figured out what was wrong with me and how to treat it.

While at Hopkins I was visited by a number of pulmonologists, oncologists, and neurologists, who ran the full gamut of tests on me to figure out what was causing my breathing problems. One of the first things they did was test my breathing capacity, which was down to 20 percent of normal. Another set of tests they wanted to perform would place me in the MRI machine for three and a half hours. This had me more than a little concerned. Lying still for that long would be difficult under any circumstances; given my reduced breathing capacity, it was next to impossible. The care team told me not to worry; they planned to hook me up to a continuous positive airway pressure (CPAP) machine attached to an oxygen tank and put me to sleep during the MRI. A CPAP machine (which is commonly used to treat sleep apnea) helps one breathe by gently pushing air into the lungs. With the CPAP and oxygen, the MRI went as planned.

On my fourth day in the ICU, after what already seemed like an endless series of tests, the doctors shared with me the list of possible diseases they were investigating. It was an ominous and frightening collection of illnesses, which included brain cancer, lung cancer, and amyotrophic lateral sclerosis (ALS), to name a few. None of these diseases has a great survival rate. However, it was the ALS that terrified me the most. ALS paralyzes voluntary muscles, which would eventually leave me unable to speak, eat, drink, or move. Not a pleasant or dignified way to spend what might be my last days on Earth.

I was still having a lot of difficulty breathing, especially at night. To help with this, the care team had me sleeping on my back with the bed raised to a thirty-five-degree angle and provided me with a CPAP machine that was attached to an oxygen tank. I usually slept on my stomach, so this took some getting used to. Breathing was only marginally better during the day. However, the care team told me that if I maintained perfect posture—back straight, shoulders back, head up, and stomach unrestrained—it would help me breathe. I did my best, but I was still hovering around 20 percent of lung capacity.

On the seventh day in the ICU, the long ordeal of testing finally ended, and I met with my physicians to hear their diagnosis. I tried my best to relax and control my growing anxiety, which I knew would only make it harder to breathe. The diagnosis began with a review of what they had eliminated, which included brain tumors, ALS, and lung cancer. While my breathing difficulties had forced me to keep a good posture, I somehow managed to sit up even straighter in response to this great news. However, my excitement was about to slump.

According to my doctors, I had an extremely rare disease called Parsonage-Turner Syndrome (PTS)—named after two British neurologists, Maurice Parsonage and John Turner, who identified and studied the disease in the 1940s. PTS typically attacks the brachial plexus, which is a network of nerves that extends from the spinal cord through the neck, connecting the brain with the chest, shoulder, arm, forearm, and hand.

PTS is an autoimmune disease, which meant that my body's own immune system had for some reason attacked these nerves. Those with PTS usually suffer damage to the nerves that control the arm and hand, and in fact my left arm was a bit atrophied, indicating some nerve damage. However, in this case the PTS had primarily affected the phrenic nerve, which controls the diaphragm. With my phrenic nerve thus affected, my diaphragm was for the most part inactive. Therefore, I only had the muscles in my rib cage and stomach to power my lungs. This was why my breathing was so limited.

I took a moment to digest this devastating new information and add it to my already grim cancer diagnosis. I then asked the obvious question, "How do we treat it?"

There was a long pause, and then I was told that, given how rare this disease is, it was not clear why my immune system had attacked my phrenic nerves, how to stop the disease from progressing, or how to restore these nerves so that I could breathe normally. It was not just the experts at Johns Hopkins who were in the dark about PTS; the medical community at large knew little about this puzzling disease, nor were there any effective treatments.

What they did know was that of the nineteen cases of PTS for which they had reliable data, about a third got better, a third did not improve, and a third got worse. Because most patients don't show any change in the first six months after diagnosis, it would likely take at least that long before I'd know where I stood. Even if I was among the lucky 33 percent who got better, it might take years before my nerves totally regenerated, and there was no guarantee that my breathing would ever be at 100 percent again.

This was good news and bad news. The good news was that the jury was still out on my chances of surviving the PTS, and the survival odds were better than fifty-fifty. The bad news was that I had only a 33 percent chance of recovering, and my breathing might never return to normal.

Of course, this was only the PTS. I also had an all-out cancer battle on my hands. When I asked how the cancer might affect my ability to overcome the PTS, the doctors told me there was no medical record of any patient fighting advanced cancer and PTS at the same time. However, they believed that the cancer should likely not affect the PTS, and the PTS should likely not affect the cancer. The truth was, given the paucity of data on PTS, nobody had any real idea how these two diseases might interact.

In the end, they recommended that I take advantage of the professional counseling that Hopkins offers for patients with severe or terminal diseases and told me they were discharging me in the afternoon.

This was quite a load to bear. However, I thanked the team, exchanged some handshakes, and they left my ICU room. As the door closed, I tried to grasp what I was facing. Two realities weighed heavily on my mind—the tough odds of beating each disease and how difficult it would be to beat both of them at the same time. I'm not a gambler, but I'd say the combined odds would be a hell of a long shot in Vegas.

> " It doesn't matter what I've gone through. There's always somebody who has had it worse than me. "
>
> —DAVID GOBIN, A PERSON WITH CANCER

The PTS was clearly the more puzzling of the two diseases I faced. To what extent did the 33 percent recover? How bad did it get for the 33 percent who got worse? What was my life going to be like if my condition stayed the same? If I did recover, could PTS come back to haunt me later? I could only conclude that my doctors and I would be learning together as we moved forward. One thing was for sure: if radiation and hormonal therapy did not get the cancer under control in the next six months, I'd be in serious trouble, regardless of PTS.

I was once again facing tough odds filled with uncertainty. It would have been easy at this point to finally throw in the towel. I mean how much can one body take? I had advanced prostate cancer and was struggling to breathe from a disease nobody knew how to cure. Either one of these could easily kill me. To make things even worse, around that same time, my doctors also informed me that I had osteoporosis. Things were clearly going from bad to worse.

> **CAREGIVER STORY:** *Vonda Cowling*

Vonda Cowling and her daughter, Trina Taylor, lived close to each other in Baltimore City and saw each other quite often. Vonda says that during the winter of 2012, Trina lost a lot of weight, found blood in her stool, and was subsequently diagnosed with colorectal cancer. She was only thirty-eight years old.

Trina's cancer was very aggressive. After numerous attempts to combat it with chemotherapy, surgeons performed an extensive surgery, which removed her spleen, her ovaries, part of her liver, her colon, and her rectum. She would need to have a colostomy bag for the rest of her life.

Trina's cancer and its complications put a large strain on her relationship with her husband, and they separated, which sent Trina into a deep depression. Vonda says that Trina asked her, "Is it because I have this colostomy? Is it because I have cancer? I'm unattractive, I know. Nobody else is going to want me."

Not long after that, Vonda got a strange text from Trina that simply said, "I love you." Trina's stepmother also got a similar strange text and called Vonda to ask her if she had recently seen Trina.

Vonda lived only five minutes away from Trina and had a key to her house. She rushed over and found Trina's father and step-mother already there. They had rung the bell, to no avail. Vonda let them in, and they called for Trina. They received no reply, so they went up to her bedroom door. It was locked, but her father broke the door down. They found Trina lying unresponsive on her bed, but still breathing. She had taken an overdose of pills.

Her parents called an ambulance and Trina was taken to the hospital, where she recovered and was admitted to the psychiatric unit. As terrifying as that was, Vonda says that suicide attempt really turned things around for Trina.

"Once she got out of the psych ward, she was a changed person. She told me, 'This is day one, and I'm choosing happy.' She chose happy, and she was happy. As a matter of fact, she said to me that 'You're not going to believe this, but even though I have cancer, this is the happiest I have been in my whole life.'" Vonda says Trina's whole demeanor and everything just changed; it was as if she had a completely new life. She had made up her mind that she wanted to live and be happy, and that's how she spent the rest of her life.

Vonda says Trina was a tall, beautiful woman, and she always showed up for her chemotherapy treatments dressed to the nines, wearing five-inch stilettos. "She was five feet, ten inches tall, so with those heels she was well over six feet and a force to be reckoned with." Everybody on the cancer unit at Johns Hopkins Hospital got to know her. Trina would talk to the other women and try to boost their spirits by giving them fashion tips and telling them they are beautiful in spite of cancer. She even started putting money aside to buy little gifts for people she knew who were on chemotherapy.

"She had this extraordinary strength, and this attitude I didn't even know she had in her. I had absolutely no idea. You know they say you never know how you're going to react to something until it happens to you."

Vonda says Trina started a group called the Osto Beauties with three other young women who had also undergone ostomies (see Sources Cited, Osto Beauties 2019). They started going out to various different community events and hospitals, reaching out to other people who had or were getting ostomies and telling them what to expect.

Trina had done a little modeling in her teens, and it had always been her dream to continue along that path. In 2015, that dream came true. She got a call from a fashion designer who had heard about Trina and the Osto Beauties and asked her to model for New York Fashion Week. After that, Trina got a number of modeling jobs, which even included a trip to Paris.

Word of Trina's great success in the face of all she had undergone started to create a buzz, and she made several TV appearances and was invited to participate in the televised fundraiser *Stand Up To Cancer* in Los Angeles, where she met various Hollywood celebrities. "Everything that she asked for at that point happened for her; it was amazing."

Sadly, in January of 2018, cancer finally caught up with Trina, and her health deteriorated rapidly. Three months later, Trina made the decision to stop treatments and enter hospice care at home. "We had a little gathering, and she had a lot of her friends there, and I and all my sisters were there, and Trina told us, 'I've been doing all this and fighting for you all, but what I'm doing now is for me.' There were people at that gathering I'd never met before who told me, 'You just don't know how your daughter has helped me.' One woman who had breast cancer said, 'Your daughter would call me to check on me, to see how I was doing, because I was getting ready to start chemo.' Another woman said, 'When I had chemo I was a basket case. But Trina would tell me to make sure I do my hair, to make sure I put lipstick on and dress up for chemo. Trina would tell me that it's only one day, get through it, and then face the next day. Your daughter kept me alive.'"

Chapter 15

WITH MY PROSTATE CANCER growing and Parsonage-Turner Syndrome limiting me physically, I was facing a lot, but did my best to keep my spirits up and remain hopeful. My post-surgery period of healing was almost over, and I started preparing for my upcoming radiation treatments at Johns Hopkins in Baltimore.

Given that I would have five sessions of radiation treatments per week for nine weeks and some important projects to attend to as the new chairman of the board of Johns Hopkins Medicine, I decided to find a place to stay in Baltimore for the duration of my treatments. This would also give me the opportunity to look into other ways to help support Hopkins as part of my ongoing desire to have meaningful purpose in my life.

Before beginning these sessions, I met with the radiation team in the basement of the Weinberg Building, where they kept this rather large machine that I would get to know very well over the next couple of months. The team explained that each daily treatment session would last approximately thirty minutes. I would have to lie flat and motionless, and it was very important that I didn't miss any sessions.

I explained to them that I had PTS and needed a CPAP device to breathe, and that it would be difficult for me to lay flat for thirty minutes. I asked if it was possible to adjust the machine to a thirty-five-degree incline. They told me the CPAP device was not a problem, but lying at an incline would not work. They suggested that over the ensuing weeks before treatment, I practice lying flat and completely still with the CPAP mask until I could manage it comfortably for thirty minutes. We shook hands, and I left with my new assignment.

Back at home in Connecticut, I started practicing with the CPAP machine for my radiation treatments. I began with short sessions at thirty degrees, gradually increasing the length of these sessions and lowering the incline until I was able to lie flat for an extended period of time. Thanks to this "training" period, the radiation treatments went surprisingly well.

Around this time, I got the courage to ask Dr. DeWeese what he thought my chances were of surviving prostate cancer. He told me I had roughly a fifty-fifty chance of living cancer free for five years. He qualified his statement by saying this was just an estimate, as there was no way to be sure. No matter how he couched it, it was grim news. These odds were worse than what I'd faced with my leukemia battle, and they did not even take into account my PTS.

While I tried to keep my spirits up, lying on the radiation table for thirty minutes, five days a week for nine weeks left a lot of room for thought, and my thoughts were a familiar bundle of uncertainties. Will the radiation and hormonal therapy eliminate my cancer? Will they prevent the cancer from spreading? If the treatments fail, are there any other viable options? Will I survive my PTS? How will PTS affect my cancer, and vice versa?

With all this uncertainty and doubt spinning through my head, I found myself thinking about the very meaning of life and once again seriously considering the possibility of death. Is there really life after death? Did God hear my prayers? Have I appropriately thought through my estate plan? If the rest of my life is short, how do I best live it?

If Dr. DeWeese was right, and I only had a 50 percent chance of living cancer free for five years, what could I do to maximize the impact of my remaining years? I had progressively stepped up my "purpose" by increasing my financial contributions to help support Johns Hopkins Medicine and also provide assistance to the disadvantaged. However, I still wanted to do more. This "purpose" was not only a welcome distraction from all my medical concerns; it also helped fuel my determination and hope while keeping despair at bay.

Call it another epiphanic moment, but during those many hours of cancer treatments, coupled with a very uncertain lung disease and advanced osteoporosis, I came to a conclusion. Instead of just giving a portion of our savings and investments to help the disadvantaged, Anne and I should give most of it away. We would keep a reasonable amount for our children and grandchildren as an inheritance, but we would donate most of our net worth to projects that advance medicine, help the disadvantaged, and hopefully make this world a better place.

I ran the idea past Anne, and we spent days talking it through. In the end, we agreed that helping others brought meaningful purpose to our lives and was an impactful way to spend the rest of our time on Earth.

> " I don't dwell on what cancer did to me. It's what cancer has done for me. And it has done a lot for me. "
> —DAVID GOBIN, A PERSON WITH CANCER

My work at Hopkins had introduced me to the groundbreaking research they were doing with stem cells and molecular biology, specifically how we could use this new science to treat cancer. Anne and I were so inspired by this work and what it could mean to the future of cancer treatments, we eventually decided to endow a chair to support research in these fields of study. The endowed chair would pay much of the salary and a portion of research costs of a chosen faculty member whose work in stem cells and molecular biology showed great promise.

Today, that chair is occupied by Professor Gregg L. Semenza, director of the Vascular Program in the Johns Hopkins Institute for Cell Engineering. Dr. Semenza discovered a key protein that allows cancers to survive in low-oxygen environments. His work is so important and novel, it earned him the coveted Lasker Award in 2016 and the Nobel Prize in 2019.

In addition to funding Dr. Semenza's work, I also later got involved in the development of Johns Hopkins University School of Medicine's new curriculum. This was long overdue, as the curriculum had not been fundamentally restructured in more than ninety years—a time span that has seen ever-evolving new technologies and the need for increasingly complex levels of interdisciplinary teamwork. Gone are the days of the solitary physician traveling from patient to patient armed only with his simple black "doctor's bag" of knowledge. Today's medicine requires the collaboration of technicians, nurses, physicians, and specialists with a wide range of professional abilities to deliver the appropriate care. For medical education to be effective and current, it must accurately reflect and teach to this new paradigm.

As one might imagine, retooling the curriculum at Hopkins Medicine was a huge undertaking, which required a special task force of the institution's top professors, researchers, and leaders. It took this group of brilliant minds five years to research and design the new curriculum, which they called Genes to Society. This exciting new curriculum embraced state-of-the-art science and technology, which digitalized labs, made lectures interactive, and promoted team learning. It literally redefined how Johns Hopkins taught medicine.

I met with the task force on numerous occasions throughout the process. One of the big concerns that came up at these meetings was whether the institution's current medical education building—a sixty-year-old structure—would be suited for the new technologies and team-oriented nature of the new curriculum. Anne and I discussed this matter and decided to make one of our largest donations to help create a new medical education building that would support and enhance this exciting new curriculum.

The promise of expanding my purpose did much to help keep my mind off the long tedious weeks of radiation therapy. When my nine-week-long treatment sessions in the Hopkins basement finally came to an end, and it was time to return to Connecticut, I was happy to be going home, but my life was far from "back to normal." My PSA numbers remained high, I still suffered from osteoporosis, and my breathing was limited and labored due to the PTS.

Regardless, I hoped for the best, and Anne and I again began to discuss our game plan going forward. For a time frame, we focused on the next few years; there were too many unknowns to plan any farther into the future. Taking a positive approach, we assumed that I'd suffer no new diseases, my cancer would stay under control or diminish, my bones would get stronger, and my breathing would stay manageable or perhaps even improve. With this relatively healthy outlook under our belts, we agreed on two courses of action. First, we'd continue to expand on our plan to give back to help others. Second, we'd find new ways to enjoy life as much as possible.

Part of enjoying life involved starting to accept social invitations again. One that came our way was an invitation to a cocktail and dinner party from a very nice couple we were quite fond of and hoped to get to know better. At the party, much to our surprise, they asked if we would like to join them on a three-week trip to New Zealand. The trip included a week on a cruise ship that would take us around New Zealand with daily ports of call, followed by an additional two weeks of traveling within the country. This was just what we needed to pick up our spirits and get our minds off of metastasizing cancer, PTS, and osteoporosis. We were not sure, however, if this trip was even possible, particularly given my breathing problems. We thanked them very much for inviting us and said we'd get back to them.

To make this trip a reality, I had to address a number of health issues, especially my PTS. At night, I was dependent on a CPAP machine with oxygen and needed to sleep on my back at a thirty-five-degree angle. This generated some potentially significant issues. How would my breathing be affected by a pressurized airplane cabin? How would I sleep in so many different accommodations? Could I survive a power outage? Would I be able to engage in some of the more strenuous activities that were planned along the way? Was it wise to be so far removed from the physicians who were the most familiar with my care? What if something went seriously wrong and I got worse? What would my doctors say about a trip of this magnitude? In spite of all these doubts, we agreed to remain positive and try to make this work. We began checking off the boxes of all that needed to be done for me to safely travel to New Zealand.

First, I got the airline's permission to take my CPAP device and a box of oxygen canisters with me in the cabin. I also looked into purchasing a back-up CPAP device and several long-lasting batteries, just in case we found ourselves somewhere with limited or no access to electricity. My biggest challenge, however, was how to breathe comfortably and sleep all night at an angle less than thirty-five degrees. The likelihood that each of our accommodations would have an adjustable bed was pretty much zero.

To address this, I once again began practicing sleeping flat on my back as I had done for my radiation treatments. Only this time I'd need to be able to breathe comfortably for much longer than thirty minutes. To help with this, I allowed for a modest "pillow incline," which I assumed I could easily arrange in my various accommodations abroad. After a few weeks of rigorous training, I got more or less used to the arrangement and was confident that we could safely make the trip to New Zealand.

When I asked my doctors about the trip, they were a bit incredulous. However, after explaining our quite extensive and successful preparations, they gave a reluctant "okay." We immediately accepted the invitation from our friends to join them.

During the ensuing months, something else unexpectedly wonderful happened. With the continuing hormonal therapy, my PSA count was slowly moving to "negligible." Dr. DeWeese cautioned that while the cancer appeared to be diminishing, we still had a few years of hormonal shots and PSA testing ahead of us. However, I still saw this news as a significant milestone in my cancer battle that was worth celebrating. As we looked forward to our impending voyage, we felt like we were not only leaving the country but also leaving my cancer behind.

Of course, there was still the PTS. However, with a good supply of oxygen canisters, an oxygen machine, two CPAP devices and back-up batteries, I was prepared. All of this weighed over eighty pounds and required two additional very large bags, but it was essential to help ensure that this wonderful trip didn't become a life-threatening event.

As the date of our much-needed New Zealand vacation grew closer, we got some great news. One morning, about three weeks before the trip, I woke up to discover that I wasn't wearing my CPAP mask, which had somehow come off during the night. At first I was troubled, and then I was elated. I had slept soundly through the night without any trouble breathing. The next evening I went to bed without either the CPAP machine or oxygen and again slept the entire night with no issues. I was actually breathing on my own!

I called the team at Hopkins and they concluded that my phrenic nerves must be regrowing. They told me to come to Hopkins as soon as possible to have my breathing tested and my phrenic nerves examined.

The very next day I went to Baltimore, and to my surprise and joy, the doctors at Hopkins confirmed that my phrenic nerves were reconnecting my brain to my diaphragm, and my breathing had improved from 20 percent to 70 percent of normal. My PTS was on the mend! Miraculously, I was one of the 33 percent who get better. I asked my doctors about the trip to New Zealand and whether I should take all the breathing equipment. They told me it would probably be all right to leave it behind, but the decision was mine.

The doctors also gave me more good news. In addition to my cancer moving toward remission and marked improvements in my breathing, the osteoporosis was at bay and my bones were getting stronger. That meant I'd likely be able to take full advantage of all the activities that awaited us in New Zealand.

When I returned from Baltimore, I continued to sleep without the CPAP and oxygen to make sure it was safe to leave them behind. I also increased my level of walking, biking, and swimming. To my inexpressible excitement and relief, I didn't feel tired, nor did I have any significant shortness of breath. Thus, Anne and I decided there was no need to drag all the heavy cumbersome "breathing" gear to the other side of the world. With all this great news, it was still premature to think that my cancer and PTS had been totally cured. However, it was amazing that I was actually boarding a plane to New Zealand in relatively good health.

As we had hoped, the trip went flawlessly. I was able to participate in all the outings and activities we had on our calendar and had no issues sleeping at night. More importantly, getting back to a "regular" routine did enormous things to help boost my spirits and take my mind off of the endless tests and treatments that I suffered with my cancer and other diseases.

Not long after that fantastic trip to New Zealand, I went to see Dr. DeWeese to get an update on my cancer, PTS, and osteoporosis. After some tests he told me that my cancer was "under control," my lung capacity was up to 87 percent, and the osteoporosis was gone. He also said that instead of having a 50 percent chance of living cancer free for five years, I now had an 80 percent chance of living cancer free for ten or more years.

Needless to say, this new prognosis went far beyond my expectations. Only months before that meeting with Dr. DeWeese, I had literally been fighting for my life on a number of fronts. Not only that, but as I write this book fifteen years later, I remain cancer free.

Epilogue

CANCER CATEGORICALLY CHANGED my perception of life and my role in it. It opened my eyes to many new opportunities for supporting medical research and inspired me to act meaningfully to help people in need.

Many of us have a desire to do something extraordinary, something selfless, that helps make this world a better place. However, we often run out of time before we have the chance to do something about it. The basic necessities of life fill up our days, weeks, months, and years, and then, often without much warning, life ends before we get a chance to discover what could be our bigger purpose.

Cancer changes that. It forces us to consider mortality sooner than we might ever have expected. This awakening has a powerful effect on our outlook on life. In my case, it inspired me to try to improve the world by assisting people who were less fortunate than I and by supporting medical research and education.

Throughout the years since I recovered from my cancers, my purpose has continued to expand to include a number of rewarding and exciting programs. One of these involved two very close friends whom Anne and I had gotten to know in Naples, Florida, Ken and Lois Werner, who have dedicated their lives to improving the living conditions of poor Maya villagers in Guatemala.

There are more than a hundred Maya villages in this mountainous region of Guatemala, with a total population of roughly ninety thousand. Most villages are small, families average six to ten people, and almost all fathers work in the fields, earning only six to eight dollars a day. The homes consist of two- to three-room huts built from corn stalks, and the kitchens have a hole in the ground with a grate over it for a stove with no chimney. The rainy season lasts four to five long months, leaving six to ten family members crammed inside these smoky little huts.

Through the Werners' nonprofit organization, People for Guatemala, I have been involved in helping Ken and Lois with a number of projects to improve conditions for these villagers, including providing food and fresh running water, establishing a health clinic, and building schools. In addition to my financial contributions, I also make regular trips to this region of Guatemala to work with the Werners, defining and designing some of the organization's many projects. One of the greatest joys of those visits is seeing how much our work is helping these good-natured, religious, and grateful people.

Another organization (a little closer to home) that I support is the Neighborhood Health Clinic (NHC) in Naples, Florida, which was started in 2008 by Dr. Bill Lascheid and his wife, Nancy, a nurse. The clinic provides medical services for working people without health insurance who have an income below two times the poverty level. I was shocked to learn that more than fifty thousand people in Collier County, Florida, meet this criterion. The NHC has a medical and dental team of more than three hundred volunteer doctors and nurses supported by some two hundred volunteer citizens. For those patients requiring specialized treatment or in-patient surgery, NHC has developed relationships with the local hospitals and health care providers.

In addition to these and other activities, I continue to support medical research and other programs at Johns Hopkins Medicine. One area that piqued my interest was the exciting and emerging field of patient safety. Up to ninety-five thousand patients die from preventable medical harm in the United States alone (see Sources Cited, Hogan et al. 2015). In spite of Johns

Hopkins' efforts to improve its safety record, like most hospitals, it was still struggling.

The institution had successfully improved its safety record in one area of care—prescription errors—but it still needed to address preventable harm related to infections, diagnosis, medical devices, tests, operating rooms, hygiene, discharge, and handoffs, to name just a few. If we tried to tackle these areas one at a time, it would take far too long. We needed a central, integrated body whose primary goal would be to research, educate, and collaborate on ways to mitigate harm across all Johns Hopkins' hospitals.

In 2011, after much fact-finding and many meetings, Anne and I donated the necessary funding to create the Armstrong Institute for Patient Safety and Quality, an integral part of Johns Hopkins Medicine. Today, the Armstrong Institute is not only actively reducing medical errors and preventable harm across all Johns Hopkins hospitals, it has also established itself as a national and global leader in patient safety.

Cancer caused me a lot of anxiety and uncertainty, but it also enabled insights and new levels of awareness that I might never have experienced if it were not for my disease. I can't say I'm glad I had cancer, nor do I want it to return, but perhaps everything happens for a reason.

What I can say is this: in spite of the many challenges cancer brought into my life, it also taught me how much more I can do with my life. And for that, I am thankful.

Acknowledgments

Over the years that I struggled with my two cancers, and during the time I spent researching this book, I've met a number of fascinating clinicians, researchers, and fellow patients. These encounters proved instrumental in helping me better understand the complexities and mysteries of cancer and the many emotional and physical challenges patients face dealing with this terrible disease. I therefore chose to include a collection of stories and insights I'd gained from these encounters, and I would like to both thank and acknowledge these clinicians, researchers, and patients for their essential contributions.

First and foremost, I owe a special debt of gratitude to the feverish work of the many dedicated, hard-working clinicians and researchers who devote their lives to better understanding and treating cancer. Their efforts and contributions have helped extend lives and increase hope for millions of patients.

While I firmly believe that hope and purpose can have a positive effect on the cancer journey, survival depends primarily on excellent diagnosis, treatment, and care. If it had not been for medical research and the great work of my two primary cancer physicians, Dr. Robert Peter Gale and Dr. Ted DeWeese, I likely would not have survived either my leukemia or my prostate cancer.

We are in an exciting time now; many new developments and technologies are helping us better understand, treat, and possibly even cure cancer. While I cannot begin to cover the entire scope of global cancer research, I can provide here a brief glimpse of some of the emerging scientific discoveries that are providing hope and promise to the field of cancer.

Two researchers who are doing great work finding better ways to detect cancer early are Dr. Nikolas Papadopoulos, at

Johns Hopkins University School of Medicine, and Dr. Ben Ho
Park, at Vanderbilt University Medical Center.

One concept that has great potential is something called
"liquid biopsies." As body cells die, they are discharged into
the bloodstream. If a person has cancer, DNA from these discharged cells should theoretically show up in the blood. New
screening technology is making it easier to detect and identify
DNA in blood, which makes diagnosing cancer by means of
liquid biopsies a potential reality.

If liquid biopsies work and are affordable, we could get a full-
body cancer screen via a blood test during our annual checkup.
This test would not only identify cancer before it grows and
spreads but would also tell us what kind of cancer we are dealing
with, enabling us to target it with the right treatments.

Another researcher I'd like to recognize is Dr. William Matsui, at the University of Texas at Austin, who is doing groundbreaking work studying cancer stem cells.

Nearly all the cells in our body have a relatively short life
span; they are born, perform a function, and then die. Tissue-
specific stem cells (also known as adult, or somatic, stem cells)
have the very special job of replacing dying cells with new cells.
Researchers now believe that cancers also have tissue-specific
stem cells; this could explain why some cancers recur and grow
so quickly. Many cancer treatments focus on killing cancer cells,
not cancer stem cells. However, scientists believe that just fo-
cusing our efforts on attacking regular cancer cells is potentially
futile, because cancer stem cells can quickly replace them.

Scientists are now looking for new drugs that will also attack
and kill cancer stem cells. One approach that is currently in
clinical trials combines bone marrow transplants (BMTs) with
an antibody that targets and kills blood cancer stem cells as a
possible cure for some forms of blood cancer.

One of the most exciting and promising areas of research
that is producing real-time results is immunotherapy. Some of

the top leaders in that field are Drs. Elizabeth Jaffee, Suzanne L. Topalian, and Stephen B. Baylin, at Johns Hopkins University School of Medicine. Cancer is an "invasive" disease: cancer cells are mutated cells that don't normally exist in our body. As such, our body should identify them as foreign and attack and kill them, as with any other "infection." However, cancer is also an "evasive" disease, which finds ways of hiding from our immune system. The goal of immunotherapy is to help the body's natural immune system better identify cancer cells, attack, and kill them.

There is great promise in this field, and the results are already evident. Immunotherapy works effectively (a year or more of remission) in about 20 percent of many cancers. In melanoma, immunotherapy is extending remission to ten years and in some cases even longer.

An additional brilliant researcher who has significantly advanced the science of cancer treatment is Dr. Richard J. Jones at Johns Hopkins University School of Medicine. His work in BMT has effectively made this life-saving treatment available to a much larger group of patients.

Bone marrow creates many of the important immune system cells that we need to survive. The bone marrow (and thus the immune system) of patients with lymphoma or other blood-related cancers often gets damaged from chemotherapy and radiation treatments. A BMT injects a healthy donor's bone marrow and immune cells into the bone marrow of a cancer patient, strengthening the recipient's immune system so that they can safely endure the treatments they so desperately need to fight cancer.

Traditionally, BMTs required a matching donor, which is not always easy to find. If the donor does not match, the donor immune cells can attack the recipient's healthy cells. This is a serious and potentially life-threatening condition, one that causes a range of medical problems. However, researchers have discovered new therapies that greatly reduce this risk, therefore opening the door to a much wider pool of donors. Researchers are also looking at ways to expand the science of BMTs to treat selective organ cancers.

In addition to thanking these and other clinicians and researchers for their hard work finding new ways to treat cancer, I also want to acknowledge the many brave cancer patients I've met along the way whose stories provide both inspiration and hope.

Cancer took center stage in my life, directing every aspect of my actions and decisions. Throughout this epic and often challenging saga, I have encountered a varied cast of other cancer patients reading from a similar script. One key story line we all share is the need to find hope and purpose to help manage cancer and all its associated challenges. This is evident across a wide range of experiences, touching people from all walks of life. Through these shared experiences, we learn that no matter how difficult our struggle, we are not alone, there is always hope.

I extend thanks and gratitude to the following clinicians, patients, and researchers who helped me write this book.

- Dr. Nilofer Azad, Associate Professor of Oncology, Sidney Kimmel Comprehensive Cancer Center at the Johns Hopkins Medical Institutions (JHMI)

- Dr. Stephen B. Baylin, Virginia and D. K. Ludwig Professor of Oncology and Medicine; Co-Director, Cancer Genetics and Epigenetics Program, Sidney Kimmel Comprehensive Cancer Center, JHMI

- Dr. Julie Brahmer, Professor of Oncology; Co-Director, Upper Aerodigestive Disease Program at the Bloomberg-Kimmel Institute for Cancer Immunotherapy, Sidney Kimmel Comprehensive Cancer Center, JHMI

- Vonda Cowling, mother of Trina Taylor, who had colorectal cancer

- Dr. Theodore DeWeese, Sidney Kimmel Professor of Radiation Oncology and Molecular Radiation Sciences, Urology, and Oncology; Vice Dean for Clinical Affairs and President of the Clinical Practice Association, JHMI

- Anna Ferguson, Senior Oncology Research Nurse, Sidney Kimmel Comprehensive Cancer Center; founder and Director, Johns Hopkins Hope Project, JHMI

- Dr. Robert Peter Gale, Visiting Professor of Haematology, Centre for Haematology Research, Department of Immunology and Inflammation, Imperial College London, London, UK

- David Gobin, former Baltimore City police officer who has lung cancer

- Christine Hogdon, person with breast cancer who is a metastatic breast cancer advocate

- Dr. Elizabeth Jaffee, Dana and Albert "Cubby" Broccoli Professor of Oncology; Deputy Director, Sidney Kimmel Comprehensive Cancer Center; Co-Director, Skip Viragh Center for Pancreatic Cancer, JHMI

- Dr. Richard J. Jones, Professor of Oncology and Medicine; Director, Bone Marrow Transplantation Program, JHMI

- Gillian Brooke Lichota, founder and Chief Executive Officer, iRise Above Foundation

- Dr. William Matsui, Professor of Oncology, Dell Medical School, University of Texas at Austin; Deputy Director, LIVESTRONG Cancer Institutes

- Jill Mull, breast cancer survivor, Johns Hopkins Breast Cancer Patient Navigator and Health Educator, JHMI

- Dr. William Nelson, Professor of Oncology; Marion I. Knott Director, Sidney Kimmel Comprehensive Cancer Center, JHMI

- Dr. Nikolas Papadopoulos, Professor of Oncology, JHMI

- Dr. Ben Ho Park, Professor of Medicine; Director, Precision Oncology, Vanderbilt University Medical Center

- Leslie S. Ries, attorney, breast cancer survivor and cofounder of the John Fetting Fund for Breast Cancer Prevention, JHMI

- Dr. Thomas Smith, Professor of Oncology, Sidney Kimmel Comprehensive Cancer Center; The Harry J. Duffey Family Professor of Palliative Medicine; Director, Palliative Medicine, JHMI

- Dr. Vered Stearns, Professor of Oncology; Director, Women's Malignancies Disease Group, Breast Cancer Research Chair in Oncology, JHMI

- Dr. Suzanne Topalian, Bloomberg-Kimmel Professor of Cancer Immunotherapy; Professor of Surgery and Oncology; Director, Melanoma Program, Sidney Kimmel Comprehensive Cancer Center; Associate Director, Bloomberg-Kimmel Institute for Cancer Immunotherapy, JHMI

Resources

1. Map and List of National Cancer Institute–Designated Cancer Centers, by State
2. Questions to Ask Your Doctor and Care Team
3. Trusted Websites on Cancer
4. Trusted Websites on Clinical Trials for Cancer
5. Managing Cancer and Work
6. Trusted Websites on Cancer Support
7. Trusted Websites on Cancer and Hope

RESOURCE 1.
Map and List of NCI-Designated Cancer Centers, by State

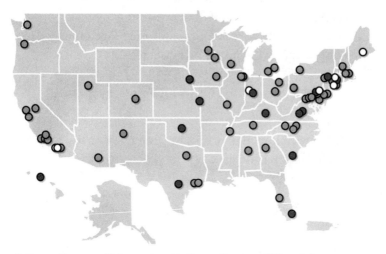

● Cancer Center   ◉ Comprehensive Cancer Center   ○ Basic Laboratory

This map of the United States indicates the location of the three different types of NCI-designated cancer centers: basic laboratory cancer centers, cancer centers, and comprehensive cancer centers. (National Cancer Institute: www.cancer.gov /research/infrastructure/cancer-centers/find/.)

According to the National Cancer Institute website, NCI-designated cancer centers divide into three categories: basic laboratory cancer centers, cancer centers, and comprehensive cancer centers.

Basic laboratory cancer centers are primarily focused on laboratory research and often conduct preclinical translation while working collaboratively with other institutions to apply these laboratory findings to new and better treatments. These centers generally do not provide patient care, although they might be able to direct you to a center that does.

Cancer centers are institutions that conduct cancer research and also provide patient care. They are recognized for their scientific leadership, resources, and the depth and breadth of their basic, clinical, and/or prevention cancer research.

Comprehensive cancer centers provide all that you would find at a cencer center. However, they provide an added depth and breadth of research, as well as substantial transdisciplinary research, which bridges different scientific areas.

The map indicates the location of each type of center (see Sources Cited, NCI, Find a Cancer Center 2019).

NCI-Designated Cancer Centers, by State

Alabama
- O'Neal Comprehensive Cancer Center, University of Alabama at Birmingham

Arizona
- Arizona Cancer Center, University of Arizona, Tucson

California
- Chao Family Comprehensive Cancer Center, University of California, Irvine, Orange
- Stanford Cancer Institute, Stanford University, Stanford
- City of Hope Comprehensive Cancer Center, Duarte
- UC Davis Comprehensive Cancer Center, University of California, Davis, Sacramento

- Jonsson Comprehensive Cancer Center, University of California, Los Angeles
- Moores Comprehensive Cancer Center, University of California, San Diego, La Jolla
- Salk Institute Cancer Center, La Jolla
- UCSF Helen Diller Family Comprehensive Cancer Center, University of California, San Francisco
- Sanford Burnham Prebys Medical Discovery Institute, La Jolla
- USC Norris Comprehensive Cancer Center, University of Southern California, Los Angeles

Colorado
- University of Colorado Cancer Center, Aurora

Connecticut
- Yale Cancer Center, Yale University School of Medicine, New Haven

District of Columbia
- Georgetown Lombardi Comprehensive Cancer Center, Georgetown University, Washington

Florida
- Moffitt Cancer Center, Tampa
- Sylvester Comprehensive Cancer Center, University of Miami, Miller School of Medicine, Miami

Georgia
- Winship Cancer Institute, Emory University, Atlanta

Hawaii
- University of Hawaii Cancer Center, Honolulu

Illinois
- Robert H. Lurie Comprehensive Cancer Center, Northwestern University, Chicago

- University of Chicago Medicine Comprehensive Cancer Center, Chicago

Indiana
- Melvin and Bren Simon Cancer Center, Indiana University, Indianapolis
- Purdue University Center for Cancer Research, West Lafayette

Iowa
- Holden Comprehensive Cancer Center, University of Iowa, Iowa City

Kansas
- University of Kansas Cancer Center, University of Kansas, Kansas City

Kentucky
- Markey Cancer Center, University of Kentucky, Lexington

Maine
- Jackson Laboratory Cancer Center, Bar Harbor

Maryland
- Sidney Kimmel Comprehensive Cancer Center, Johns Hopkins University, Baltimore
- Marlene and Stewart Greenebaum Comprehensive Cancer Center, University of Maryland, Baltimore

Massachusetts
- Dana-Farber/Harvard Cancer Center, Boston
- David H. Koch Institute for Integrative Cancer Research at MIT, Massachusetts Institute of Technology, Cambridge

Michigan
- Barbara Ann Karmanos Cancer Institute, Wayne State University School of Medicine, Detroit
- Rogel Cancer Center, University of Michigan, Ann Arbor

Minnesota
- Masonic Cancer Center, University of Minnesota, Minneapolis
- Mayo Clinic Cancer Center, Rochester

Missouri
- Alvin J. Siteman Cancer Center, Washington University School of Medicine and Barnes-Jewish Hospital, St. Louis

Nebraska
- Fred and Pamela Buffett Cancer Center, Nebraska Medicine and the University of Nebraska Medical Center, Omaha

New Hampshire
- Norris Cotton Cancer Center at Dartmouth, Dartmouth-Hitchcock Medical Center, Lebanon

New Jersey
- Rutgers Cancer Institute of New Jersey, Rutgers Biomedical and Health Sciences, New Brunswick

New Mexico
- University of New Mexico Cancer Research and Treatment Center, University of New Mexico, Albuquerque

New York
- Albert Einstein Cancer Center, Albert Einstein College of Medicine, Bronx
- Memorial Sloan-Kettering Cancer Center, New York City
- Cold Spring Harbor Laboratory Cancer Center, Cold Spring Harbor
- Roswell Park Comprehensive Cancer Center, Buffalo
- Herbert Irving Comprehensive Cancer Center, Columbia University, New York City
- Tisch Cancer Institute, Icahn School of Medicine at Mount Sinai, New York City
- Laura and Isaac Perlmutter Cancer Center, New York University Langone Health, New York City

North Carolina

- Duke Cancer Institute, Duke University Medical Center, Durham
- Wake Forest Baptist Comprehensive Cancer Center, Winston-Salem
- UNC Lineberger Comprehensive Cancer Center, Chapel Hill

Ohio

- Case Comprehensive Cancer Center, Case Western Reserve University, Cleveland
- Ohio State University Comprehensive Cancer Center, James Cancer Hospital and Solove Research Institute, Columbus

Oklahoma

- Stephenson Cancer Center, University of Oklahoma, Oklahoma City

Oregon

- Knight Cancer Institute, Oregon Health and Science University, Portland

Pennsylvania

- Abramson Cancer Center, University of Pennsylvania, Philadelphia
- UPMC Hillman Cancer Center, Pittsburgh
- Fox Chase Cancer Center, Philadelphia
- Wistar Institute Cancer Center, Philadelphia
- Sidney Kimmel Cancer Center at Jefferson, Thomas Jefferson University, Philadelphia

South Carolina

- Hollings Cancer Center, Medical University of South Carolina, Charleston

Tennessee
- St. Jude Children's Research Hospital, Memphis
- Vanderbilt-Ingram Cancer Center, Nashville

Texas
- Dan L Duncan Comprehensive Cancer Center, Baylor College of Medicine, Houston
- Mays Cancer Center at UT Health San Antonio, University of Texas Health Science Center, San Antonio
- Harold C. Simmons Comprehensive Cancer Center, University of Texas Southwestern Medical Center, Dallas
- University of Texas MD Anderson Cancer Center, Houston

Utah
- Huntsman Cancer Institute, University of Utah, Salt Lake City

Virginia
- Massey Cancer Center, Virginia Commonwealth University, Richmond
- University of Virginia Cancer Center, Charlottesville

Washington
- Fred Hutchinson/University of Washington Cancer Consortium, Seattle

Wisconsin
- University of Wisconsin Carbone Cancer Center, Madison

RESOURCE 2.
Questions to Ask Your Doctor and Care Team

It's a good idea to copy these questions (and any others you have) and bring them along with you when you see your doctor.

- What type of cancer do I have?
- What is the stage of my cancer?
- Has it spread to other areas of my body?
- Will I need more tests before treatment begins? Which ones?
- Will I need a specialist for my cancer treatment?
- Will you help me find a doctor for a second opinion on the best treatment plan?
- How serious is my cancer?
- What are my chances of survival?
- What are the ways to treat my type and stage of cancer?
- What are the benefits and risks of each of these treatments?
- What treatment do you recommend? Why do you think it is best for me?
- When will I need to start treatment?
- What is my chance of recovery with this treatment?
- How will we know if the treatment is working?
- Would a clinical trial (research study) be right for me?
- How do I find out about studies for my type and stage of cancer?
- Where will I go for treatment and how is it given?
- Will I need to be in the hospital for treatment? If so, for how long?
- How many treatment sessions will I have and how long will each take?
- Should a family member or friend come with me to my treatment sessions?
- What side effects may occur during or between my treatment sessions?

- Are there any lasting effects of the treatment?
- How can I prevent or treat side effects?
- Are there any side effects that I should call you about right away?
- Could any medicines or dietary supplements I am taking change the way that cancer treatment works?

(See Sources Cited: NCI. Questions to Ask Your Doctor about Cancer. 2019.)

RESOURCE 3.
Trusted Websites on Cancer

The information on each of the following websites has been vetted by top cancer physicians and researchers. You can also find reliable information on the websites of NCI-designated cancer centers. Finally, there are some nonprofit patient advocacy websites that also contain valuable information and resources specific to your disease. Important to note, any and all data you derive from the internet should be cross-checked and cross-referenced to ensure that it comes from a reputable and reliable source, and then it should be reviewed by your care team.

- American Cancer Society. (See Sources Cited: ACS. 2019.)
- American Society of Clinical Oncology. (See Sources Cited: Cancer.Net. 2019.)
- National Cancer Institute. (See Sources Cited: NCI. 2019.)
- National Comprehensive Cancer Network. (See Sources Cited: NCCN. 2019.)
- Society for Integrative Oncology. (See Sources Cited: SIO. 2019.)

RESOURCE 4.
Trusted Websites on Clinical Trials for Cancer

Listed here are a number of reputable websites that can help you find clinical trials that might work for you. You can also look on the websites of NCI-designated cancer centers and the websites of properly vetted, nonprofit organizations specific to your disease. Just make sure to cross-check and cross-reference all data you get from these sites and run everything past your care team.

- American Cancer Society: How Do I Find a Clinical Trial That Is Right for Me? (See Sources Cited: ACS. How Do I Find a Clinical Trial That Is Right for Me? 2020.)
- National Cancer Institute: Steps to Find a Clinical Trial. (See Sources Cited: NCI. Steps to Find a Clinical Trial. 2019.)
- National Comprehensive Cancer Network: Find a Clinical Trial. (See Sources Cited: NCCN. Find a Clinical Trial. 2020.)
- National Institutes of Health. (See Sources Cited: NIH. ClinicalTrials.Gov. 2019.)
- U.S. Food and Drug Administration: Clinical Trials. (See Sources Cited: FDA. Clinical Trials. 2019.)

RESOURCE 5.
Managing Cancer and Work

The nonprofit organization Cancer and Careers is an excellent resource dedicated solely to helping cancer patient manage work and all the challenges associated with cancer. It provides legal advice, financial advice, cancer coaches, information about events and other activities, and advice on managing co-workers and time off for treatments. (See Sources Cited: Cancer and Careers. 2020.)

The many websites and organizations listed in this Resources chapter also have additonal information and support to help patients balance work and cancer.

You should also ask your employer what services and support they offer cancer patients.

An example of an employer-sponsored program is Managing Cancer at Work, which is available at Johns Hopkins Medicine, Nissan, Novartis, AARP, Latham & Watkins, Gonzaga University, Pitney Bowes, Quest Diagnostics, the Vitamin Shoppe, and Church's Chicken. (See Sources Cited: WorkStride. 2020.)

RESOURCE 6.
Trusted Websites on Cancer Support

In addition to the specific resources listed above, I have listed some additional websites here that provide general support to cancer patient family members and caregivers.

- American Cancer Society: Treatment and Support. (See Sources Cited: ACS. Treatment and Support. 2019.)
- CancerCare. (See Sources Cited: CancerCare. 2019.)
- Get Palliative Care. (See Sources Cited: Get Palliative Care. 2019.)
- National Cancer Institute: Cancer Support Groups. (See Sources Cited: NCI. Cancer Support Groups. 2019.)
- National Comprehensive Cancer Network: Advocacy and Support Groups. (See Sources Cited: NCCN. Advocacy and Support Groups. 2019.)

RESOURCE 7.
Trusted Websites on Cancer and Hope

Cancer clinicians, researchers, and other caregivers are beginning to embrace the important role hope plays in the cancer experience. I have listed a few websites here that provide specific resources and compelling patient stories regarding hope and purpose in the face of cancer. You should also ask your care team what resources they have to help you find and maintain hope and purpose in your journey through cancer.

- American Cancer Society: Stories of Hope. (See Sources Cited: ACS. Stories of Hope. 2019.)
- Cancer*Care*: Stories of Help and Hope. (See Sources Cited: Cancer*Care*. Stories of Help and Hope. 2019.)
- Cancer Hope Network. (See Sources Cited: CHN. 2019.)
- Hope Matters. (See Sources Cited: JHMI. Hope Matters. 2019.)

Glossary

Atrophied. Having wasted away or decreased in size (as from disease or disuse).

B Cells. A key component of the adaptive humoral immune system, these cells mediate the production of antigen-specific immunoglobulin (antibodies) directed against invasive pathogens.

Bilateral. Of, relating to, or affecting the right and left sides of the body or the right and left members of paired organs.

BRCA1 Mutation. A gene on chromosome 17 that normally helps to suppress cell growth. A person who inherits certain mutations (changes) in a BRCA1 gene has a higher risk of getting breast, ovarian, prostate, and other types of cancer.

Cancer Stages. Stage 0 means abnormal cells are present but have not spread to nearby tissue; also called carcinoma in situ, or CIS. CIS is not cancer, but it may become cancer. Stages 1–3 mean cancer is present. The higher the number, the larger the cancer tumor and the more it has spread into nearby tissues. Stage 4 means the cancer has spread to distant parts of the body.

Clinical Trials. Clinical trials are research studies, performed in people, that evaluate a behavioral, surgical, or medical intervention. They are the primary method researchers use to discover whether a new treatment (e.g., drug, diet, or medical device) is effective and safe for humans.

Colostomy. Surgical formation of an artificial anus by connecting the colon to an opening in the abdominal wall.

CPAP. A continuous positive airway pressure ventilator for people who can breathe spontaneously on their own but need some assistance.

Immunotherapy. Treatment or prevention of disease (such as an autoimmune disorder, allergy, or cancer) that involves the stimulation, enhancement, suppression, or desensitization of the immune system.

Mastectomy. Surgical removal of all or part of the breast and sometimes associated lymph nodes and muscles.

Metastasis. The spread of a pathological agent (such as cancer cells) from the initial or primary site of disease to another part of the body.

Parsonage-Turner Syndrome. A disease that attacks a network of nerves called the brachial plexus, which control movement and sensation in the shoulders and arms. While the cause is still unknown, PTS is believed to be related to an autoimmune response following exposure to an illness or environmental factor. Treatment generally focuses on symptoms and may include corticosteroids, pain relievers, and physical therapy.

Placebo. An inert or innocuous substance used especially in controlled experiments testing the efficacy of another substance (such as a drug).

PSA Test. A blood test that measures the level of a protein (prostate-specific antigen) produced by the prostate gland. PSA blood levels are often elevated in men with prostate cancer.

Remission. A decrease in or disappearance of signs and symptoms of cancer. In partial remission, some, but not all, signs and symptoms of cancer have disappeared. In complete remission, all signs and symptoms of cancer have disappeared, although cancer still may be in the body.

Tissue-Specific Stem Cells. Also known as adult stem cells, or somatic stem cells, these cells are found throughout the body and can divide to replenish dying cells and regenerate damaged tissues. They are found in children as well as adults. Tissue-specific stem cells, unlike embryonic stem cells, are often restricted to certain cell lineages, whereas embryonic stem cells can theoretically become any cell in the body.

Triple Negative Breast Cancer. Triple negative breast cancer lacks the three most common types of receptor known to fuel most breast cancer growth—estrogen, progesterone, and the HER2/neu gene. Thus, common treatments, such as hormone therapy and drugs that target estrogen, progesterone, and HER2, are ineffective.

Sources Cited

ACS (American Cancer Society). www.cancer.org. Published 2019.

ACS. How Do I Find a Clinical Trial That Is Right for Me? www.cancer.org/treatment/treatments-and-side-effects /clinical-trials/what-you-need-to-know/picking-a-clinical -trial.html. Published 2019.

ACS. Prostate Cancer. www.cancer.org/cancer/prostate-cancer .html. Accessed 2020.

ACS. Stories of Hope. www.cancer.org/latest-news/stories-of -hope.html. Published 2019.

ACS. Survival Rates for Pancreatic Cancer. Cancer A-Z website. www.cancer.org/cancer/pancreatic-cancer/detection -diagnosis-staging/survival-rates.html. Published 2019.

ACS. Treatment and Support. www.cancer.org/treatment /support-programs-and-services. Published 2019.

Cancer and Careers. www.cancerandcareers.org/en. Published 2019.

Cancer*Care*. https://www.cancercare.org/. Accessed 2020.

Cancer*Care*. Stories of Help and Hope. www.cancercare.org /stories. Published 2019.

Cancer.Net. American Society of Clinical Oncology. www.cancer.net. Published 2019.

CHN (Cancer Hope Network). www.cancerhopenetwork.org. Published 2019.

FDA (U.S. Food and Drug Administration). Clinical Trials: What Patients Need to Know. www.fda.gov/patients /clinical-trials-what-patients-need-know. Published 2019.

Ferrell BR, Temel JS, Temin S, et al. Integration of Palliative Care into Standard Oncology Care: American Society of

Clinical Oncology Clinical Practice Guideline Update. *Journal of Clinical Oncology.* 2017;35(1):96–112.

GetPalliativeCare. Get Palliative Care. www.getpalliativecare .org. Published 2019.

Hogan H, Zipfel R, Neuburger J, et al. Avoidability of hospital deaths and association with hospital-wide mortality ratios: retrospective case record review and regression analysis. *The BMJ.* 2015;351.

Hope Matters, Johns Hopkins Medical Institutions. www.hopkinsmedicine.org/kimmel_cancer_center /centers/hope_matters/. Published 2019.

NCCN (National Comprehensive Cancer Network). www.nccn.org. Published 2019.

NCCN. Advocacy and Support Groups. www.nccn.org /patients/advocacy/. Published 2019.

NCCN. Find a Clinical Trial. www.nccn.org/patients/resources /clinical_trials/find_trials.aspx. Published 2019.

NCCN. Phases of Clinical Trials. NCCN. Patient and Caregiver Resources website. www.nccn.org/patients/resources /clinical_trials/phases.aspx. Published 2019.

NCI (National Cancer Institute). www.cancer.gov. Published 2019.

NCI. Cancer Support Groups. www.cancer.gov/about-cancer /coping/adjusting-to-cancer/support-groups. Published 2019.

NCI. Find a Cancer Center. www.cancer.gov/research/nci-role /cancer-centers/find. Published 2019.

NCI. NCI-Designated Cancer Centers. www.cancer.gov /research/infrastructure/cancer-centers. Published 2019.

NCI. Questions to Ask Your Doctor about Cancer. www.cancer .gov/about-cancer/coping/questions. Published 2019.

NCI. Steps to Find a Clinical Trial. www.cancer.gov/about -cancer/treatment/clinical-trials/search/trial-guide. Published 2019.

NIH (National Institutes of Health). ClinicalTrials.Gov. www.clinicaltrials.gov. Published 2019.

Osto Beauties. www.ostobeauties.com. Published 2019.

SIO (Society for Integrative Oncology). https://integrativeonc .org/patients/guide-to-credible-internet-info. Published 2019.

USGov. Family and Medical Leave Act. www.dol.gov/agencies /whd/fmla. Accessed 2020.

WorkStride. Work Stride: Managing Cancer at Work. Johns Hopkins Medicine. www.workstride.org/. Published 2019.

Index

American Society of Clinical Oncology, 41
amyotrophic lateral sclerosis (ALS), 102
antibiotics, 53, 60–61, 67, 68
Armstrong Institute for Patient Safety and Quality, 119
atrophy, 53, 75, 103, 139
AT&T, 78, 89
Aurelius, Marcus, ix–x
autoimmune diseases, 103, 140
Azad, Nilofer, 29, 124

Bakewell, Danny, 72–73
Baylin, Stephen B., 122–23, 124
B cells, 16, 139
blood tests, 83, 85, 122. *See also* PSA (prostate-specific antigen) test
bone marrow test, 14
bone marrow transplants (BMTs), 122–24
Brahmer, Julie, 10, 25, 28, 124
BRCA1 mutation, 82, 83, 139
breast cancer: and BRCA1 mutation, 82, 83, 139; patient stories of, 15, 52–54, 74–77, 81–84; treatment for, 42, 52–53, 74, 82–83; triple negative, 81–82, 141
breathing, 99–102, 115–16. *See also* Parsonage-Turner Syndrome (PTS)

cancer: emotional aspects of, 13, 19, 74–75, 77; as "invasive" disease, 123; metastasized, 15, 29, 93, 140; prevention, 83–84; undetected, 12–13, 16; websites on, 22–23, 135. *See also* breast cancer; colorectal

cancer; leukemia; lung cancer; pancreatic cancer; prostate cancer
Cancer and Careers (nonprofit organization), 136–37
cancer stages, 26–27, 139
cancer support: for breast cancer patients, 77; for lung cancer patients, 97–98; from nurse/ patient navigators, 40; from palliative care team, 40–41; from patient navigators, 40, 41–43; and support groups, 42, 97, 137; websites on, 137
chemotherapy: and bone marrow transplants, 123; for breast cancer, 42, 43, 52–53, 74, 82–83; for colorectal cancer, 105, 106, 107; digestive problems from, 43; hair loss from, 43, 52, 83; for leukemia, 19, 22, 30–33, 37, 44, 49–50, 51; for lung cancer, 95; for pregnant women, 74–75
children: with cancer, 69, 71, 72–73; encounters with death by, 45, 46–47; talking to, 43
clinical trials: about, 25–26, 139; deciding to enter, 27–28; for immunotherapy, 29, 96–97; investigation of, 28–29; for Pentostatin, 16, 19–20, 28; phases of, 26–27; side effects from, 26, 27, 33, 96; websites on, 136
Clostridium difficile (C. diff) infections, 53
colorectal cancer, 29, 105
colostomy, 105, 139
Cowling, Vonda, 105–7, 125

ABOUT THE AUTHORS

Under President Bill Clinton, **Mike Armstrong** was the chairman of the President's Export Council, the U.S.-Japan Business Council, and the FCC's Network Reliability and Interoperability Council. He was also a member of the US Business Council and the Business Roundtable, where he served as the chairman of homeland security. In addition, he served as a member of the National Security Telecommunications Advisory Committee and the Defense Policy Advisory Committee. He was a visiting professor at the MIT Sloan School of Management. He is a member of the Council on Foreign Relations and the Conference Board.

Eric A. Vohr worked as lead science writer for Johns Hopkins Medicine and the Endocrine Society. He is the coauthor of *Safe Patients, Smart Hospitals: How One Author's Checklist Can Help Us Change Health Care from the Inside Out*, and he is currently writing a textbook on patient safety for the Armstrong Institute for Patient Safety and Quality at Johns Hopkins Medicine. Vohr received his master's degree in creative writing from Johns Hopkins University, where he also taught science writing.